STAT!

Medical Office Emergency Manual

Jeryll A. Tuttle-Yoder

Susan A. Fraser-Nobbe

Notice to the Reader

Publisher does not warrant or guarantee any of the products described herein or perform any independent analysis in connection with any of the product information contained herein. Publisher does not assume, and expressly disclaims, any obligation to obtain and include information other than that provided to it by the manufacturer.

The reader is expressly warned to consider and adopt all safety precautions that might be indicated by the activities described herein and to avoid all potential hazards. By following the instructions contained herein, the reader willingly assumes all risks in connection with such instructions.

The publisher makes no representations or warranties of any kind, including, but not limited to, the warranties of fitness for particular purpose or merchantability, nor are any such representations implied with respect to the material set forth herein, and the publisher takes no responsibility with respect to such material. The publisher shall not be liable for any special, consequential or exemplary damages resulting, in whole or in part, from the readers' use of, or reliance upon, this material.

Cover Credit: Robyn Eskenazi-Gray

Publishing Team:
Publisher: David C. Gordon
Acquisitions Editor: Marion Waldman
Project Manager: Helen Yackel

Editorial Assistant: Sarah Holle
Project Editor: Melissa A. Conan
Art and Design Coordinators: Vincent S. Berger
and Richard Killar

COPYRIGHT © 1996
By Delmar Publishers
A division of International Thomson Publishing Inc.
The ITP logo is a trademark under license
Printed in the United States of America
For more information, contact:
Delmar Publishers
3 Columbia Circle, Box 15015
Albany, New York 12212-5015

International Thomson Editores
Campos Eliseos 385, Piso 7
Col Polanco
11560 Mexico D F Mexico

International Thomson Publishing Europe
Berkshire House 168-173
High Holborn
London, WC1V7AA
England

International Thomson Publishing GmbH
Königswinterer Strasse 418
53227 Bonn
Germany

Thomas Nelson Australia
102 Dodds Street
South Melbourne, 3205
Victoria, Australia

International Thomson Publishing Asia
221 Henderson Road
#05-10 Henderson Building
Singapore 0315

Nelson Canada
1120 Birchmount Road
Scarborough, Ontario
Canada M1K 5G4

International Thomson Publishing - Japan
Hirakawacho Kyowa Building, 3F
2-2-1 Hirakawacho
Chiyoda-ku, Tokyo 102
Japan

1 2 3 4 5 6 7 8 9 10 XXX 01 00 99 98 97 96 95

Library of Congress Cataloging-in-Publication Data
Tuttle-Yoder, Jeryll A.
    STAT : medical office emergency manual / Jeryll A. Tuttle-Yoder,
Susan A. Fraser-Nobbe.
        p.   cm.
    Includes index.
    ISBN 0-8273-6489-X
    1. Medical emergencies.   2. Ambulatory medical care.   3. Medical
offices.   I. Fraser-Nobbe, Susan A.   II. Title.
    [DNLM: 1. First Aid—methods.   2. Emergencies.   3. Crisis
Intervention—methods. WA 292 T967s 1995]
RC86.7.T88   1996
616.02'5—dc20
DNLM/DLC
for Library of Congress   95–14211
                                                                 CIP

Dedication

This work would not have been possible without the loving support of our families and friends, especially Jon, Kathryn, Daniel, Andrew, Gary, and Danielle, with their inexhaustible patience and encouragement.

Table of Contents

Preface

In over 25 years of experience as health educators and medical assisting instructors, it has always been necessary for us to glean essential information from a variety of sources. This text presents vital information to help medical professionals handle emergencies effectively in today's medical office setting.

It is essential for medical office personnel to be trained in emergency response techniques. The Emergency Medical System (EMS) is an effective and efficient responder in a medical crisis, but the person in medical crisis could die before the EMS arrives. To reduce the risk to the patient and increase the chances of survival and recovery, medical office personnel must be trained in emergency response techniques.

Training in emergency techniques is also necessary for:

- Dealing with an emergency calmly and efficiently. Many people panic when confronted with an emergency situation. Knowing what to do helps the responder stay calm, which in turn can influence the emotional response of the patient and/or bystanders.

- Operating within the scope of training. In an emergency, the responders need to know the boundaries of their training so that mistakes in care can be avoided and auxiliary personnel can be contacted if necessary.

- Handling situations that may be potentially harmful to the patient or others in the office. The likelihood of an emergency situation becoming uncontrolled increases if no one present is trained in emergency procedures. To decrease the potential for inappropriate action or accidents, office personnel need to be trained in handling a variety of emergency situations.

- Self care. In the event that a member of the team needs emergency assistance and no trained responder is available, it may be necessary for the health care professional to instruct an untrained person in what care to render, and how the procedure should be carried out.

- Responding to the emergency within legal guidelines. The medical professional will need to be aware of the legal guidelines concerning an emergency situation in order to decrease the possibility of litigation. Avoiding violation of these guidelines can be achieved if personnel understand the legal implications of their actions.

Appropriate training and effective procedural guidelines allow office personnel to respond in an authoritative and knowledgeable manner, thus calming those directly and indirectly involved in an emergency situation.

Basic first-aid training needs to be obtained from a universally recognized organization such as the Red Cross. The Red Cross offers a wide variety of programs, including first-aid training, cardiopulmonary resuscitation (CPR), and basic life support (BLS). Appropriate training is also available through various community organizations. Medical office personnel should explore the training programs available in their community. The importance of a training program that adequately prepares office professionals to deal with emergencies cannot be overemphasized.

Text features include:

- Objectives at the beginning of each chapter.
- Logical information sequencing.
- Cross-referencing.
- User-friendly text.
- Coverage of legal aspects as they pertain to emergency situations and professional responsibility.
- Information on the principles and application of psychological first aid techniques for emergencies.
- Information on assembling a crash cart/drawer.
- Review questions stressing critical thinking scenarios.

Appendices include DACUM Guidelines, OSHA's Blood-Borne Pathogen and Universal Precaution Guidelines, Frequently Used Telephone Numbers Form, State Agencies for Reporting Child Abuse and Neglect, State Aging and Adult Protective Service Agencies, and a Glossary.

Text highlights are:

- Telephone response guidelines that include questions, responses, actions to be taken, and rationales for office use.
- Information concerning stress and burnout along with management techniques for the health care professional.
- Chapters on some of today's most prevalent concerns: helping victims of abuse and neglect as well as helping the abuser.
- Instructor's Guide that includes activities, critical thinking scenarios, and discussion questions to facilitate the learning process.

The procedures presented in this text are not intended to provide an individual with training in CPR, rescue breathing, or choking; rather they are to be used as a quick reference for individuals already trained. Everyone should have formal training in these areas.

Acknowledgements

From the very beginning, this book has had input and assistance from a variety of people. We would especially like to thank Charles Carroll and Fred Evans for their support and advice; Gary Macdonald, Charles Butcher, Gary Clapp, Misty Kirby, and Chris Wagner for their help with the photography; Linda Pruitt, Ann Bick, and Carolyn Yates for their typing assistance; Marion Waldman, Helen Yackel, and Sarah Holle for being so helpful and easy to work with; and our students, who gave us the inspiration for this book.

CHAPTER 1

Universal Precautions

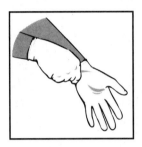

Objectives

After completing this chapter the learner should be able to:

1. Define blood-borne pathogens.
2. Define body fluids.
3. List the procedures, in correct sequence, for dealing with body fluid spills.
4. List the personal protective equipment (PPE) recommendations for the health care provider.
5. Describe the key elements of using PPEs.
6. Describe the importance of using universal precautions.

Introduction

This section presents the universal precautions that the Occupational Safety and Health Administration (OSHA) mandates all employees observe when dealing with body fluids. It is strongly recommended that every health care worker become familiar with all aspects of OSHA's regulations and rules concerning blood-borne pathogens (Appendix B). In addition, each health care facility should have an exposure control plan that will familiarize the employee with facility rules on handling body fluids.

Blood-borne Pathogens

Blood-borne pathogens are disease-causing organisms present in body fluids that can be transmitted by blood or other potentially infectious materials coming into direct contact with non-intact skin or mucous membranes, or through indirect contact by touching or handling contaminated items or surfaces.

Of the many blood-borne pathogens, human immunodeficiency virus (HIV) and hepatitis B virus (HBV) are the two that concern health care providers most. The majority of occupational HIV transmissions have occurred by accidental sticks with contaminated sharps. Special precautions should be taken by health care workers who deal with sharps. Approximately 8,700 health care workers contracted hepatitis in 1992, and about 200 will die. In comparison, as of 1991, only 84 of the estimated 200,000 AIDS patients were health care workers with no identified reason for infection. With an estimated 1.25 million potentially HBV-infected individuals in America, health care workers should consider receiving the vaccine for hepatitis B.

It is the responsibility of medical personnel to follow the guidelines for prevention of the spread of these diseases. These guidelines apply to blood, semen, vaginal secretions, cerebrospinal fluid, synovial fluid, fluid with visible blood, unidentifiable body fluid, and saliva from dental procedures.

Universal precautions protect the health care worker from contracting a blood-borne disease. In addition, patients and the families of health care workers are protected.

The need for infection control cannot be overemphasized. Every health care provider has a responsibility to use universal precautions. All body fluids should be treated as if they were known to contain HIV, HBV, or other blood-borne pathogens.

OSHA Regulations

Regulations from OSHA include gloving, masking, donning aprons, or using protective face shield or goggles whenever a worker might be exposed to blood or other potentially infectious fluids. While each facility will have its own rules, basic guidelines should not be overlooked or ignored, such as wearing latex gloves and/or covering whenever there is a risk of exposure to blood or other body fluids. When in doubt, the health care worker should wear gloves, protective face shield or goggles, apron, and lab coat (see Figure 1-1). Occasionally

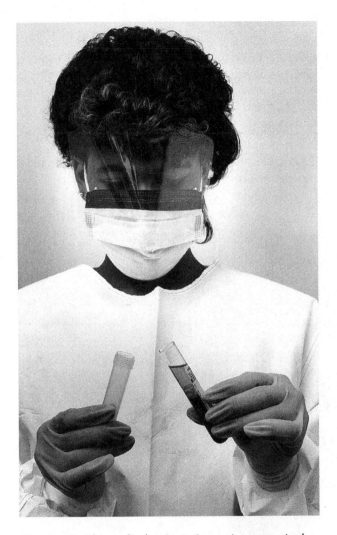

Figure 1-1   This medical assistant is wearing protective barriers: latex gloves, gown, face shield, and mask as she prepares to pour serum from a centrifuged blood tube to the transfer tube for laboratory analysis. (From Krebs and Wise, *Medical Assisting, Clinical Competencies,* © 1994, Delmar Publishers.)

patients are offended by what they consider to be "full riot gear." The sensitive health care worker will be quick to explain that the personal protection equipment protects the patient as well as the worker. Each member should also be fully versed in the correct method for cleaning spills or vomitus.

Contaminated Spill Cleanup

Cleaning a contaminated spill should be done following existing OSHA guidelines (see Figure 1-2). The basic steps are as follows:

1. Wear protective gloves and/or personal protective equipment.
2. Flood the area with bleach solution (1 part bleach to 10 parts water; only effective for 24 hours).
3. Using a dustpan and brush, clean up any broken glass. Place the glass in appropriate puncture-proof containers (sharps container—see Figure 1-3).

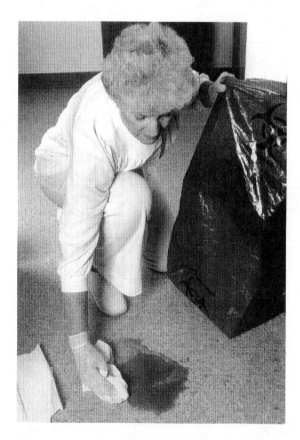

Figure 1-2   This medical assistant is wearing latex gloves to clean up a specimen spill. The biohazard waste bag is used to dispose of the contaminated materials. (From Krebs and Wise, *Medical Assisting, Clinical Competencies,* © 1994, Delmar Publishers.)

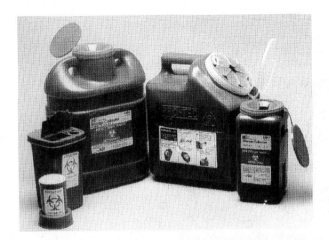

Figure 1-3 A few of the various sizes of biohazard puncture-proof containers are displayed (they are bright red and yellow to alert caution). Biohazardous waste containers must be autoclaved when full and returned to the biohazard area for proper disposal. (From Krebs and Wise, *Medical Assisting, Clinical Competencies,* © 1994, Delmar Publishers.)

4. Clean the area with paper towels or a broom and dustpan.
5. Place used towels in red biohazard bags (see Figure 1-4).
6. Remove gloves; pull them off inside out.
7. Place the gloves in the biohazard bag and tie the bag.
8. Wash hands with disinfectant soap and water for at least 10 seconds.

Importance of Personal Protective Equipment (PPE)

Every office faces the possibility of an emergency involving body fluids, which creates a legal responsibility to train staff to protect themselves and the patient adequately. Too often personnel use the excuse that there is not time to don gloves or other PPE when faced with an emergency, but emergency rooms throughout the country have no problem using protective barriers for themselves and their patients. Each office or facility should drill in the importance and actual use of universal precautions. Each office member should think it second nature to grab at least a pair of gloves. Easy access to these materials is the key element. Boxes of gloves should be located in every room of the health care facility. Additional PPE should be easily accessible if determined it is needed.

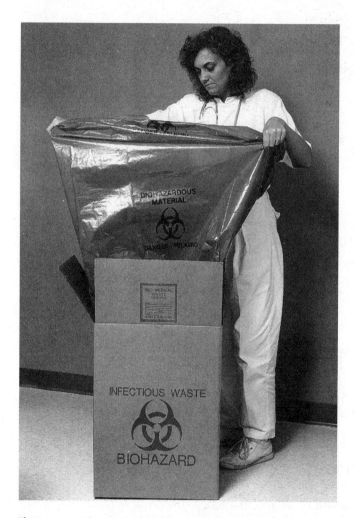

Figure 1-4   This medical assistant is placing a sturdy disposable bag marked with the biohazardous waste symbol in a durable cardboard box marked the same for collection of infective waste material. When full, these boxes are picked up by an agency for incineration or for autoclaving and disposal in a public landfill. (From Krebs and Wise, *Medical Assisting, Clinical Competencies,* © 1994, Delmar Publishers.)

The extra seconds taken to apply gloves and other PPE can protect the health care workers, their families, and even the patient.

Occasionally emergencies arise that require respiratory resuscitation. Mouth-to-mouth is not a safe practice. These emergencies should be handled with CPR microshields and resuscitation bags. The use of these devices is explained in Chapter 2.

Summary

As of 1993, it was estimated that 1 in 250 persons in the United States is infected with HIV. Individual health care workers have a legal and moral responsibility to follow OSHA's blood-borne pathogen guidelines, even in an emergency. The number of persons infected with blood-borne pathogens is expected to grow. Health care workers should remember that the greatest risk of blood-borne pathogens is from hepatitis B. Therefore, health care workers should receive the hepatitis-B vaccine.

Review Questions

1. Universal precautions were developed by what federal agency.
2. Define blood-borne pathogen as it relates to the use of universal precautions.
3. Why is the health care worker at more risk of contracting HBV?
4. List at least four body fluids and potential situations that could lead to contamination.
5. Why are facility rules on handling body fluids important?
6. When would personal protective equipment (PPE) not be appropriate?

CHAPTER 2

Emergency Procedure Guide

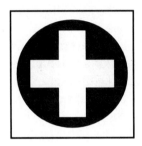

Objectives

After completing this chapter the learner should be able to:

1. List the common respiratory aids that should be maintained on a stocked emergency cart.
2. List the necessary IV supplies that should be maintained on a stocked emergency cart, as well as the function of those supplies.
3. List the medications described in the text, as well as their uses.
4. Define the chain of command.
5. List 5 standard emergency directions.
6. Define a primary survey.
7. Describe how a secondary survey is conducted.
8. Define standing orders.
9. Define triage and explain its purpose.

Introduction

In recognition of the importance that each individual deserves the best possible care, it is essential to develop and maintain an office emergency procedure guide. When developing the emergency procedure guide, it will be necessary for the office to identify who will be in charge, and what each individual's role will be. In order to be effective, this chain of command must be decided before an emergency occurs, allowing a confident and calm approach to the emergency by all of the office personnel. All office personnel should review the guidelines periodically so that procedures can be recalled without hesitation.

Precious time is often wasted as office personnel search for needed emergency equipment, only to find that the materials have expired or are not available. An emergency cart, fully stocked and checked weekly, can mean the difference between life and death for some patients. Because emergencies do happen in the medical office, it is the responsibility of each person in the office to know what to do. All members of the team will need to familiarize themselves with the supplies and equipment located on the emergency cart, know where the equipment is stored, and feel secure in their role in dealing with emergency situations.

Respiratory Emergency Aids

Because respiratory emergencies are life-threatening, it is essential to address those situations first. Respiratory aids to include on a fully stocked cart are:

- A full oxygen tank with flowmeter and attached wrench for opening the tank. Time should be taken to train personnel in the appropriate procedure for cracking the tank and adjusting the flowmeter to the instructed setting. Personnel should also be trained in administering oxygen.
- A set of airways of various sizes for maintaining an open breathing passage in the patient. In each office, adjustment needs to be made for patient size and/or age (see Chapter 6 for procedures).

For the protection of the office personnel as well as the patient, an oral barrier should be utilized when administering rescue breathing.

Oxygen can be delivered in a variety of ways. One of the most commonly used devices is the bag valve mask. The bag is capable of holding between 1300–1500 ml of air. A one-way valve allows for a direct flow of air to the patient. The mask should have an air-cushioned rim for a tighter seal to the patient's face. The bag valve mask should be equipped with an oxygen inlet for attachment to the oxygen tank. All members of the team should practice using the bag valve mask to ensure proper ventilation of the patient.

Resuscitation masks are available in a variety of sizes and models. Masks should have an inlet for the delivery of supplemental oxygen and be fitted with a one-way valve for releasing a person's exhaled air. They should be easy to assemble.

The nasal cannula (NC) is a plastic tube with two small prongs inserted into the nose. The nasal cannula is attached to an oxygen source. NCs are most often used for individuals having only minor breathing difficulty, or if the patient cannot tolerate a mask.

The venturi mask fits over the mouth and nose and has an adjustable strap much like the simple mask. However, the venturi mask allows for greater accuracy in administering oxygen. The percentage of the oxygen administered can be controlled by either a rotating opening or color-coded adapters.

The two types of airways used are oropharyngeal, inserted in the mouth, and nasopharyngeal, inserted through the nose. These airways do not pass through the larynx. The purpose of these airways is to maintain a clear opening to the tracheobronchial tube by holding the tongue back from the pharyngeal wall. The major advantages of these devices are:

1. To maintain an open airway for the patient.
2. To allow for more effective ventilation for the patient.

The equipment must be clean and the correct equipment and size will need to be selected.

IV Supplies

While it is the responsibility of the physician to establish an IV line, all members of the team should be familiar with the procedure and equipment for starting an IV. Expiration dates of IV solution should be checked on a weekly basis (see Figure 2-1).

Medications

No medications are administered without a physician's order. It may be necessary to identify standing-order medications, those medications that can be administered in a specific set of circumstances without a verbal order from the physician. All standing orders must be in writing, kept on file, signed, and dated by the physician. In the event that any questions should arise concerning the administration of a standing-order medication, documentation can protect all individuals involved.

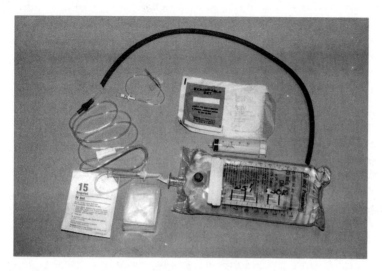

Figure 2-1   Supplies necessary to start an IV: IV solution, tubing, butterfly needle, syringe, 4 in. × 4 in. sterile gauze pads.

Medications most commonly found on an emergency cart are glucose for hypoglycemia (low blood sugar) and insulin for hyperglycemia (high blood sugar). Epinephrine and atropine are most commonly used in anaphylactic shock and cardiac emergencies. Syrup of Ipecac is used for patients who have ingested certain toxic substances in order to induce vomiting. The primary use of nitroglycerin is to treat angina pectoris (heart pain). Spirits of ammonia is used for the treatment of syncope, and normal saline is used for the cleansing of wounds. These medications and their specific uses are covered in the appropriate chapters.

All medications should be examined for expiration dates, missing labels, or discoloration every week. Outdated, unlabeled, or discolored medication should be properly disposed of. To eliminate the threat of possible misuse, medication should be flushed down the toilet with a witness present. Discarded medications should be replaced immediately.

All packages should be inspected for sterility and damage. Any damaged, outdated, or discolored supplies should be properly disposed of and replaced immediately. Two sets of batteries for the penlight should be checked weekly.

Emergency Procedure Checklist

Identified Chain of Command

- Person who witnesses the emergency alerts the appropriate personnel STAT!

- Doctor.
- Nurse.
- Medical Assistant.
- Office personnel begin patient assessment.
- Appointed personnel remains in charge until EMS personnel or physician arrives.

Stocked Emergency Cart

Emergency equipment should be stored in the emergency treatment area on a crash cart or a portable tray. Supplies to include:

Respiratory Emergency

- Oxygen tank with flowmeter and wrench for opening tank.
- Airways—all sizes; nasal and oral.
- Tubing.
- Nasal cannula.
- Mask.
- Ambu bag—adult and pediatric face mask with oxygen attachment.
- Resuscitation masks—variety of sizes.
- Bulb syringe for suction.

IV Supplies

- Butterfly needle—#19, #21, #22, #23, #25—three of each.
- Hemostat.
- Angiocath—#16, #18, #20, #22—three of each.
- Tourniquet.
- Betadine.
- Alcohol preps.
- 500 ml of D5W.
- 500 ml of NS.
- 500 ml of D10W.
- 500 ml of lactose Ringer's.
- IV tubing.
- Hammer and nails (can be used to hang an IV bag if poles are not available in the office).

Medications

- Instant glucose.
- Insulin (to be kept in the refrigerator).
- Epinephrine.
- Activated charcoal.
- Atropine.
- Lidocaine.
- Phenobarbital and diazepam.
- Sodium bicarbonate.
- Solu-Cortef.
- Verapamil.
- Xylocaine and marcaine.
- Syrup of Ipecac.
- Nitroglycerine.
- Normal saline.
- Diphenhydramine.
- Spirits of ammonia.
- Furosemide.

General Supplies

- Alcohol wipes.
- Blood pressure cuff (standard, large, pediatric).
- Stethoscope.
- Scissors (bandage).
- 4 x 4 gauze (sterile).
- Kling gauze (sterile).
- Pressure bandages—various sizes.
- Gloves—examination and sterile.
- Cravats.
- Prepackaged needles/syringes—assorted sizes.
- Hypo-allergenic tape.
- Nasogastric tube.
- Catheter tip—syringe.

- Water soluble lubricant.
- Penlight (with extra batteries).
- Hot/cold packs.
- Pen/notebook.

Standard Emergency Directions

1. Do not move the patient unless it is necessary for safety reasons.
2. Protect the patient from unnecessary manipulation and other potentially damaging factors.
3. Determine the cause of injury or sudden illness if possible. Handle any life-threatening problems.
4. Look for any emergency medical identification.
5. Examine the patient methodically, taking into consideration the kind of accident or sudden illness and the specific needs of the situation. **Have a reason for everything you do!**

Patient Assessment

1. Survey the scene.
2. Primary survey:
   - Airway.
   - Breathing.
   - Circulation.
3. Phone EMS if necessary.
4. Secondary survey:
   - Introduce yourself.
   - If the patient is conscious, get permission to give care.
   - Ask the patient's name and use it.
   - Ask the patient what happened.
   - Ask if the patient is in pain.
   - Ask if the patient is diabetic and when meals and/or medication were last taken.
   - Ask if the patient has a seizure disorder.
   - Ask if the patient is taking any medications.
   - Ask if the patient has any allergies.

- Check the patient's vital signs:
  - Pulse.
  - Respiration.
  - Blood pressure.
- Assess skin appearance, checking for color, moisture, and temperature.
- Do a head-to-toe exam if the situation and time support it.
  - Start with the head, checking for cuts, bruises, or other signs of injury.
  - Check the pupils of the eyes for size and reaction to light.
  - Check for fluid drainage from the ears, mouth, and nose.
  - Gently feel the sides of the neck to check for any pain, tenderness, or signs of injury.
  - Check and compare the collar bones and both shoulders for any signs of injury and pain.
  - Check the rib cage for signs of injury or pain, pressing firmly but gently along the sides of the chest.
  - Check the patient's abdomen for tenderness or rigidity by pressing lightly with the flat part of the fingers, checking each quadrant.
  - Check each arm, beginning at the shoulder and progressing toward the hand. Ask the patient to wiggle the fingers.
  - Press gently but firmly on the hips, checking for pain and signs of injury.
  - Check each leg, starting at the top of the leg and progressing toward the foot. Ask the patient to wiggle the toes.

If possible, move the patient to a designated treatment area. Any movement of the patient, however, needs to be based on the patient's specific condition.

Psychological First Aid

Besides paying attention to the physical needs of the patients, the health care professional must also create the right psychological atmosphere for communication with both the patient and family. The steps for good psychological first aid are:

- Remain calm. The best way to accomplish this is to know how to handle emergency situations.

- Those office personnel not directly involved in the delivery of emergency medical treatment should be tuned in to the actions and verbalization of family members and other patients in the immediate area.
- Provide emotional support to both the patient and family members.

Documentation

The patient's chart is the most important medical document during a medical emergency. The health care professional responsible for the chart should follow the steps below:

- Copies of the patient's chart should be made available to the EMS personnel.
- An incident report should be filled out immediately following the emergency. A copy of the report should be placed in the patient's chart.
- The physician should record directly onto the patient's chart all emergency procedures that were performed.

Standing Orders

The physician in charge of the office will usually write certain procedures, called standing orders, for the health care professional to follow in the physician's absence. Standing orders allow the office personnel to react to specific emergency situations in an efficient and effective way. Typical standing orders include:

- Patients in respiratory distress are typically placed on 4–6 liters of oxygen.
- Infants experiencing diarrhea and vomiting should be taken off all dairy products.
- Acetaminophen is frequently prescribed for fever and as a general pain reliever.

Triage

Triage, the French word for "sorting," is a term used by health care professionals to refer to the priorities of procedures. Whether sorting casualties by seriousness of injury after a major emergency, or determining in what order to

Table 2-1 Triage Priority Situations

First Priority	Next Priority	Least Priority
airway and breathing problems	second degree burns not on the neck and face	fractures
cardiac arrest	major or multiple fractures	minor injuries
severe bleeding that is uncontrolled	back injuries	sprains
head injuries	severe eye injuries	
poisoning		
open chest or abdominal wounds		
shock		
second and third degree burns		

treat a patient's multiple injuries, medical personnel need to develop skills in prioritizing, or triage. The main principle of triage, whether treating multiple casualties or a single patient with multiple injuries, is:

Severe bleeding and absence of breathing are immediate threats to life.

Triage of a patient with multiple injuries begins with the primary survey and continues with the secondary survey. To assist the health care professional in determining what injuries require priority treatment, Table 2-1 was developed.

Summary

First-aid training is necessary in order to facilitate appropriate patient care. Formal first-aid training is highly recommended. It will be necessary for every office to develop its own individual office emergency guide.

Review Questions

1. List 4 emergency medicines and give an example for the use for each.
2. You have found a patient unconscious in the examination room. List in sequential order the steps that you would take.

3. Describe the chain of command and give an example of where you have observed it.
4. Explain the importance of psychological first aid and what needs to take place for it to be effective.
5. Why are standing orders necessary?

CHAPTER 3

Basic Telephone Techniques and Emergency Response Guidelines

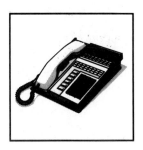

Objectives

After completing this chapter the learner should be able to:

1. Communicate effectively over the telephone.
2. Respond appropriately to callers experiencing an emergency.
3. Ask pertinent questions regarding the emergency.
4. Elicit specific information from the caller.
5. Accurately document the emergency call.
6. Effectively interact with the EMS system.
7. Refer the caller to appropriate personnel as indicated by the office guidelines.
8. Describe why a telephone response guide is necessary.
9. List six of the most common complaints heard over the phone in the medical office.
10. List pertinent questions, responses, and rationales for the conditions presented in the guideline format.

Introduction

The telephone is one of the most important means of communication that the patient has with the medical office. Because this is often the first contact the patient or patient's family has with the physician's office in a given situation, it is imperative that the individual answering the telephone be skilled in handling over-the-phone emergencies.

Basic Telephone Techniques

Answer the phone promptly. It is best to answer by the second ring. Hold the receiver 2–3 in. from the mouth to allow for proper articulation. If the person on the other end of the line cannot understand you, you will need to keep repeating yourself. Answer the phone with "Good Morning" or "Good Afternoon."

- Identify the office, for example, "Dr. Smith's office."
- Identify yourself.
- Ask who is calling and write the caller's name down.
- Respond with "How can we help you?"

After receiving information on the situation, it may be necessary to put the individual on hold. If this is the case, **ask** the individual calling if you may put the call on hold, and wait for a response before doing so. In an emergency situation, the patient needs to be able to tell the office personnel if immediate attention is required. If a patient with an emergency is put on hold, the caller might be disconnected if left on hold for an unacceptable period of time.

Always be respectful and courteous to the caller. Maintain control of the conversation by asking questions, and be sure that all information is clarified. Summarize the information and get verification from the caller that the information was understood correctly. By repeating the information back to the caller, you can avoid misunderstandings.

Decide what action needs to be taken. Every phone call that comes into the physician's office will require some action. Based on individual office guidelines and the reason for the call:

- Does the call need to be routed to someone else?
- If for the doctor, pull the chart for the doctor to have handy before taking the call.

■ Each call, whether incoming or outgoing, should be put on a message pad, and then transferred to a message log.

Individual messages should be placed in the appropriate patient file. Information that should be documented includes:

■ Current date.

■ Time of call.

■ Patient's name.

■ Patient's phone number (include extension if applicable).

■ Whom the message is for.

■ Message.

■ Action taken.

■ Name or initials of the person taking the call.

Emergency Telephone Techniques

The patient is the person who decides when there is an emergency. Because the telephone is a quick and efficient method of communication, patients will often call the physician's office first. Medical personnel need to be aware of office emergency guidelines and know what questions to ask in order to develop an individual patient's emergency action plan (Figure 3-1).

The person making an emergency call may not be calm, and may be difficult to understand. The first responsibility of the medical office personnel is to

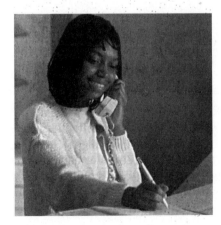

Figure 3-1 Telephone conversation (From Krebs and Wise, *Medical Assisting, Clinical Competencies,* © 1994, Delmar Publishers.)

calm the caller in order to facilitate the transfer of information. In a less agitated state, the caller will better be able to implement specific instructions.

Calming Methods

Methods for helping the caller achieve a state of calm include:

1. Maintain a calm, even, low-pitched tone of voice.
2. Use the caller's name.
3. Get the caller's attention.
4. Have the caller sit down and take 3–4 deep breaths.
5. Ask specific questions:
   - What are the patient's name and age?
   - What happened?
   - What are the signs and symptoms of injury or illness?
   - How long ago did the accident occur or symptoms begin?
   - What is being done for the patient?
   - Has the patient been on any medications? If the answer to this last question is yes, ask the name of the medication, how long the patient has been taking the medication, and if there is a possibility that the patient may be having a reaction to the medication.

Medical personnel should avoid stock phrases like "Everything will be OK." Not only is it not possible at this point to be sure that everything will be OK, but, under the law, this remark can be interpreted as a guarantee for which you could be held legally responsible. It is appropriate to tell callers that:

- They need to remain calm so that they can maintain control.
- Everything that can be done is being done.
- Emergency assistance is being summoned (if applicable).

Never diagnose The caller will often want reassurance as to what the potential problem is. Office personnel should be aware that to offer any opinion can be viewed as a medical diagnosis. Any questions should be referred to the physician and/or emergency personnel.

Emergency numbers should be posted next to all telephones in the office. Patients should be instructed as to the proper procedure for contacting the physician in an after-hours emergency. The office may want to develop a frequently used telephone number list for patients to post by their telephone at home (see Appendix C).

Frequently Used Telephone Numbers

This form should be cut down to a size suitable to be taped next to your telephone. Use the extra lines for the phone numbers of people you call frequently or may need to reach in a hurry.

If your office is outside city limits, be certain to check on what fire department to call, and whether to call the city police, state police, or county sheriff for assistance. Write down your own office address and telephone number. In an emergency, many people do not think too clearly, and a delay in assistance may be a life-or-death matter.

The form in Figure 3-2 can be used in the medical office. A copy with current phone numbers should be placed near each office phone. (A full-sized form for patients has been included in Appendix C.)

FREQUENTLY USED TELEPHONE NUMBERS	
AMBULANCE	
HOSPITAL	
POISON INFORMATION	
POLICE	
ADDITIONAL NUMBERS	
YOUR NAME	
YOUR TELEPHONE	
YOUR ADDRESS	

Figure 3-2 Sample of medical office emergency phone numbers form.

Telephone Response Procedural Guide for Patient Complaints

Panicked patients demanding help in dealing with a medical situation beyond their experience and knowledge require concise assistance from a well-prepared emergency responder. Many times the office personnel will feel inadequate and helpless when dealing with these patients. This situation need not occur! Individuals who are responsible for answering the phone and handling emergencies need to be adequately prepared. A telephone response guide can provide this assistance.

The complaints most often asked about in the office should be included in an office telephone response guide. Each problem, complete with a decision tree, should be listed and a procedural sheet developed for each potential problem. Included on the sheet should be the potential problem, a list of pertinent questions for office personnel to ask in a priority order, and actions the patient should take based on the information gathered. The physician should evaluate each potential problem to provide a set of standing orders. These standing orders are also included on the procedural sheets.

Complaints most commonly asked about over the phone are bleeding from injuries, pain, severe chest pain, poisoning, frostbite, burns, usual childhood diseases, seizures, eye injuries, animal bites, high temperatures in children, and fractures.

Monthly evaluations of the emergency telephone response guideline should be conducted to develop the most efficient instructions possible. Each procedural sheet should be examined for clear and concise direction, completeness of standing orders, and appropriateness of the selected questions. Routine inservice on individual procedural sheets should also be done. It is not enough simply to develop the emergency telephone guidelines manual; personnel must know **how** to use the information it contains.

While the process is time consuming initially, one efficiently handled telephone emergency is well worth the time and effort invested. Often, precious time is lost while office personnel notify the physician of a telephone emergency without collecting essential information for evaluation. With the creation of a procedural manual, personnel will have a reference to guide them in asking the most pertinent questions, evaluating the information gathered, and knowing when to activate the EMS without delay.

While each office must develop its own manual based on the physician's preference and office staff training, examples of the most common complaints and childhood disease procedural sheets have been developed and are included here as a guide for office use. The sheets include questions to ask, actions to take, and rationales for each action. They allow easy reference for the office when dealing with a distraught caller.

A complete list of all Response Guidelines is presented in the Table of Contents, Chapter 3.

Chicken Pox

Chicken pox is caused by a virus that also causes shingles. It is highly contagious and can be transmitted from 24 hours before the rash appears, up to 5–6 days after the first appearance of rash. It occurs primarily in young children and is spread by droplets from the mouth or throat, or by direct contact with contaminated articles. **It is not spread by dried scabs.** The incubation period is 14–21 days following the initial exposure. Usually there is fatigue and some fever 24 hours before the rash appears. The rash first appears as flat, red splotches; they become raised and resemble small pimples (see Figure 3-3). They then further develop into small blisters and form a crust consisting of dried serum. The crust flakes off in 9–13 days. Severe itching accompanies the "pustular" stage. Usually they first appear on the chest and back, then may spread to the rest of the body. There can be a few sores or hundreds. Complications are rare, but can include encephalitis and infection of the lesions.

CHICKEN POX RESPONSE GUIDE

QUESTIONS	RESPONSES	ACTION TO TAKE	RATIONALE
Is convulsion, stiff neck, severe lethargy, or headache present? NO	YES ◊	Patient to come to ◊ office immediately.	May indicate the development of encephalitis.
Are lesions surrounded by redness or draining pus? NO	YES ◊	Patient to come to ◊ office immediately.	Infection of lesions requires antibiotic therapy.
Is rapid breathing present? NO	YES ◊	Consult physician. ◊	Physician needs to evaluate the patient further.
Consult physician.			Physician has final decision whether patient is seen.

With physician approval, the following instructions may be given:

- Warm bath with baking soda to reduce the itching (1/2 cup to tubful of water).
- Antihistamines—particularly Benadryl—to relieve itching.
- Acetaminophen to relieve fever.
- Cut the patient's fingernails or have patient wear gloves to reduce the chances of infection in the lesions from scratching.

(continues)

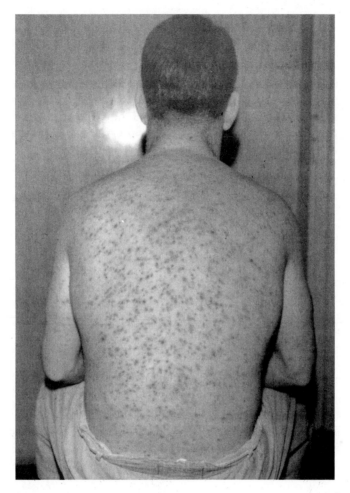

Figure 3-3 Chicken pox. (Courtesy of Armed Forces Institute of Pathology #62-12553.)

(Chicken Pox, continued)

- Hands should be washed frequently to reduce the chances of infecting the lesions.
- If lesions are in the mouth, gargle with salt water to reduce discomfort (1/2 tsp salt to 8-oz. glass).
- Advise caller to bring patient in the back or side door if coming to the office.

NOTE: Disinfect the room following the visit, using an aerosol spray, and let stand for 20 minutes before using the room again.

Rubella (German or Three-Day Measles)

Rubella is a mild viral infection spread by droplets from the mouth or throat. Signs and symptoms include mild fatigue and enlarged lymph nodes possibly occurring at the back of the neck. Incubation period is 12–23 days. The rash, characterized as flat or slightly raised red spots that quickly spread to the trunk and the extremities, first appears on the face; however, there may be no rash. The spread of the rash is highly variable. The fever rarely rises above 101°F and usually lasts less than 2 days; 15–20 percent of infected individuals experience joint pain around the third day of illness. Complications are extremely rare, but the primary concern is the infection of a fetus. Exposure during the first trimester of pregnancy can cause the development of cataracts, heart disease, deafness, and mental deficiency in the fetuses of about 50 percent of the women exposed.

RUBELLA (GERMAN OR THREE-DAY MEASLES) RESPONSE GUIDE

QUESTIONS	RESPONSES	ACTION TO TAKE	RATIONALE
Has patient experienced lethargy or convulsions? NO ⬅	YES ⟿	Patient to come to ⟿ office immediately.	Symptoms may indicate the development of complications.
Is there any bleeding or bruising? NO ⬅	YES ⟿	Patient to come to ⟿ office immediately.	May indicate the development of complications.
Has there been any contact with a pregnant woman or her children? NO ⬅	YES ⟿	Have her contact ⟿ her physician immediately.	Increased risk to the unborn child.
Consult physician.			Physician has final decision whether patient is seen.

With physician approval, the following instructions may be given:

- Acetaminophen to relieve fever.
- Warm water bath.
- Advise caller to bring patient in the back or side door if coming to the office.

NOTE: Disinfect the room following the visit, using an aerosol spray, and let stand for 20 minutes before using room again.

Rubeola (Measles)

Rubeola or measles is a viral illness that begins with weakness, fever, and a dry cough; eyes are itchy, red, and sensitive to light. The rash will follow in 3–5 days, first noticed around the hairline, on the face, on the neck, and behind the ears. It then spreads to the chest and abdomen and finally to the extremities. The rash becomes redder and larger as the disease progresses (Figure 3-4). There may be some light brown coloring to the skin lesions. The contagious time frame is 3–6 days before the rash appears, to several days after it appears. It is spread by droplets from the mouth or throat and by direct contact with contaminated articles. Symptoms appear 8–12 days after exposure to the virus. Common complications are sore throat, ear infections, pneumonia, and measles encephalitis (a serious complication that can lead to permanent brain damage).

RUBEOLA RESPONSE GUIDE

QUESTIONS	RESPONSES	ACTION TO TAKE	RATIONALE
Is lethargy, stiff neck, vomiting, headache, or convulsion present? NO ⬇	YES ↻	Patient to come to ↻ office immediately.	Symptoms of complications.
Has bleeding from nose, mouth, or rectum, or bruising of the skin, occurred? NO ⬇	YES ↻	Patient to come to ↻ office immediately.	Symptoms of developing complications.
Has patient experienced dyspnea? NO ⬇	YES ↻	Patient to come to ↻ office immediately.	Symptoms of developing complications.
Does patient complain of earache, sore throat, rapid breathing (over 40/min.)? NO ⬇	YES ↻	Patient to come to ↻ office immediately.	Symptoms of complications.
Consult physician.			Physician has final decision whether patient is seen.

With physician approval, the following instructions may be given:

- Acetaminophen to relieve fever.

(continues)

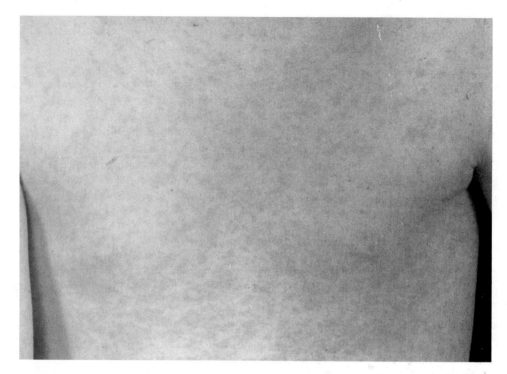

Figure 3-4   Measles on chest. (Courtesy of Armed Forces Institute of Pathology #77-21632-1.)

(Rubeola (Measles), continued)

- Vaporizer for the cough.
- Dim the lights and isolate the patient until the rash disappears.
- Advise caller to bring patient in the back or side door if coming to the office.

NOTE: Disinfect the room following the visit, using an aerosol spray, and let stand for 20 minutes before using the room again.

Mumps

Mumps is a viral infection that settles in the parotid salivary glands, but submaxillary involvement can occur. Signs and symptoms are low grade fever, headache, earache, and swelling in front of and below the ears. Mumps is contagious during the period of 6 days before the first symptom appears, to the complete disappearance of the parotid gland swelling (usually one week). Incubation period is 15–18 days after exposure. Complications can include meningoencephalitis, kidney disease, deafness, and involvement of the testicles or ovaries. Complications are rarely seen in children. While a normal progression does not require a visit to the office, it should be noted in the patient's chart.

MUMPS RESPONSE GUIDE

QUESTIONS	RESPONSES	ACTION TO TAKE	RATIONALE
Is there lethargy, convulsions, or stiff neck? NO	YES ▷	Patient to come to ▷ office.	These are classic symptoms of encephalitis.
Does the patient have any of the following: • pain and swelling of the testicles? • lightheadedness? • difficulty breathing? • abdominal pain and vomiting? NO	YES ▷	Patient to come to ▷ office.	Symptoms of the development of a complication.
Consult physician.			Physician has final decision whether patient is seen.

With physician approval, the following instructions may be given:

- Acetaminophen for pain.
- Avoid sour foods, especially orange juice (these foods make the pain worse).
- Adequate fluid intake (important to avoid dehydration).
- Adults who have not had mumps should avoid exposure.
- Advise caller to bring patient in the back or side door if coming to the office.

NOTE: Disinfect the room following the visit, using an aerosol spray, and let stand for 20 minutes before using the room again.

Poisoning

Instruct patient to call the Poison Control Center. Be sure the person calling has the bottle or example of the ingested material readily available. Instruct the person calling that the Poison Control Center is the best source for poisoning information; call the patient back for follow-up.

NOTE: Every state has a regional Poison Control Center with an 800 number. The office should post this number by each phone. Because there are a variety of substances that can cause poisoning, it is best to contact the Poison Control Center. They are the experts on all types of poisons and should always be notified for identification and treatment of a poison patient. However, every office should have Syrup of Ipecac to induce vomiting, and activated charcoal for poison absorption.

Insect Bites

Insects bites can be from bees, wasps, ticks, centipedes, and so on. It is important to ask if the caller can identify or describe the insect. Included are a general description of insects, signs and symptoms of their bites or stings, and general first-aid treatment. The guidelines are specific questions for the office staff to ask to determine if the patient needs to be seen immediately.

Spider Bites

1. Black Widow—coal-black 3/4–1 1/2 in. long. Bright red hourglass on abdomen.

   Signs and symptoms—appearance of small puncture, profuse sweating, rigid abdomen muscles, breathing difficulties, slurred speech, dilated pupils. Symptoms usually occur within 15–30 minutes.

   Treatment—patient needs immediate medical treatment.

2. Brown Recluse—brownish, rather flat, 1/2–5/8 in. long. Dark brown violin on back. Usually likes clothes, closets, and dark locations.

   Signs and symptoms—blister at site (Figure 3-5), generalized rash, joint pain, chills, fever, nausea, vomiting; pain may become severe after 8 hours.

   Treatment—ice packs slow absorption to toxin. If left untreated, toxin causes necrosis (dead tissue), and an ulcer can develop, which can take 6 weeks to heal and cause extensive tissue damage.

Scorpion Stings—straw-colored slender body of about 2 inches.

   Signs and symptoms—severe localized pain, restlessness, drooling of saliva, muscular spasms, and rapid pulse. High fever to 104°F. Labored breathing, shortness of breath. Death can occur within twelve hours.

   Treatment—constricting band should be applied about 3 inches from site for 5 minutes, then released. Pack wound with ice and transport to medical facility.

Ticks—small, flat, and oval shaped 1/8–1/4 in. long; gray or brown in color.

   Signs and symptoms—ticks attach to body and suck the victim's blood, swelling up like miniature balloons before dropping off.

   Treatment—remove ticks as quickly as possible.

   Removal method—apply substance to smother the tick such as mineral oil, vegetable oil, and so on. Lift off with tweezers after it disengages. Do not attempt to pull off. Ticks drill into the body and may snap off at the head if they don't disengage themselves.

Bee and Wasp Stings—winged body, makes buzzing sound.

   Signs and symptoms—itching and pain followed by redness and swelling at sting site. Gradually a wheal will appear, which normally subsides after a few hours.

(continues)

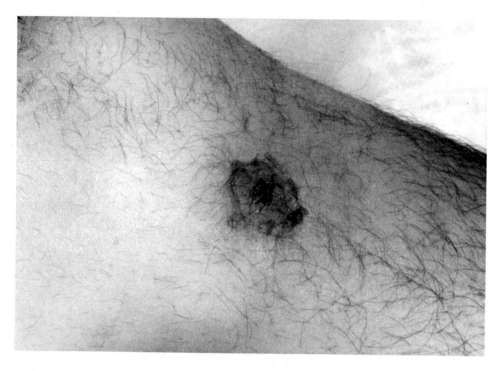

Figure 3-5   Brown Recluse Spider Bite. (Courtesy of Armed Forces Institute of Pathology #93-15395.)

(Insect Bites, continued)

However, if the following symptoms occur, seek medical attention immediately: sting is around the eyes or tongue; dry, hacking cough; sense of constriction in throat or chest; swelling and itching around eye; massive hives; sneezing. These are signs of anaphylactic shock, which is a medical emergency. Transport immediately.

Treatment—look for presence of stinger; if stinger is in the skin, scrape off with fingernails or a knife. Do not use tweezers or fingers, as this procedure breaks the venom sack and releases the venom into the wound. After examining for stingers (and removal if necessary), apply ice packs to slow absorption of toxin into the bloodstream. Wash the site with soap and water. Observe victim for signs of an allergic reaction.

(Insect Bites, continued)

INSECT BITE RESPONSE GUIDE

QUESTIONS	RESPONSES	ACTION TO TAKE	RATIONALE
Is area around the bite reddened, swollen, or itchy? YES ◆	NO ◊		
Has patient ever experienced allergic reaction to an insect bite before? NO ◆	YES ◊	Come to office ◊ immediately.	Patient is at increased risk of infection or anaphylaxis.
Is there difficulty breathing, lightheadedness, rash, or swelling present? NO ◆	YES ◊	Patient to office ◊ immediately.	Symptoms of allergic reaction.
Does bite site look infected (swollen, reddened, white patch at bite site)? NO ◆	YES ◊	Make an appointment ◊ to see the physician.	Needs medical attention.
If bite occurred over 24 hours ago, has it continued to worsen in severity? NO ◆	YES ◊	Make an appointment. ◊	Bites that continue to worsen need medical attention.
Consult physician.			Physician has final decision whether patient is seen.

Snake Bites

Snake bites rarely result in death; however, all snakes should be considered venomous. The medical professional should be aware of how to handle this type of emergency.

1. Be sure patient is removed from the area where the snake was seen, to avoid another bite.

2. Apply a constriction band above the bite area. Never apply a band around a finger or tight enough to impair arterial circulation. The band should be 3/4–1 1/2 in. wide. This band can stay on safely for one hour before it needs to be loosened, but do not release it. The band is only effective if applied within 30 minutes following the bite.

3. Apply an improvised splint if it can be done within 1–2 minutes of the bite occurring.

4. Do not allow victim to walk about. Keep victim calm.

5. If victim is over 4 hours away from a medical facility, an incision 1/4 in. long can be made in the bite and suction can be done. The preferred method is with a suction cup from a snake bite kit.

SNAKE BITE RESPONSE GUIDE

QUESTIONS	RESPONSES	ACTION TO TAKE	RATIONALE

Was the snake seen or captured?
        NO
        ⬤
	YES ◊	Take snake head to medical facility.	

Has anything been done for the victim?
        YES
        ⬤
	NO ◊	Apply constriction band ◊ (3/4–1 1/2 in. wide) above bite. This is effective only if applied within 30 minutes after bite has occurred. Keep limb in horizontal position. Do not allow victim to walk.	Retards the speed of the toxin in the bloodstream.

What was done? ⬤			
Consult physician.			Physician has final decision whether patient is seen.

Heat Emergencies

Excessive heat can affect the body in a variety of ways. In the human body, heat loss must equal heat production in order to maintain a normal body temperature. About 98.6°F (37°C) is considered to be average; slight variations from person to person are normal.

The most common heat emergencies are heat stroke (which is immediately life-threatening), heat exhaustion, and heat cramps. Because heat stroke must be dealt with immediately, the office will need to be familiar with its signs, symptoms, and treatment.

1. In heat stroke, the patient's skin is hot and red, usually dry, pupils are constricted, and the body temperature is very high. This condition is life-threatening and requires prompt action. The patient must be cooled down quickly to prevent brain damage.

2. In heat exhaustion, the patient will have cool, pale, and moist skin with heavy sweating, dilated pupils, headache, nausea, vertigo, and vomiting. The body temperature will be near normal. Treatment involves increased water intake and avoidance of sun.

3. Heat cramps involve muscular pain and spasms due to heavy exertion, usually involving abdominal muscles and the legs. It is believed to be brought about by the loss of water and salt through heavy sweating. Treat by increasing the intake of electrolytes and avoiding exercise.

Medical personnel need to keep in mind the environmental factors associated with the disorders: temperature, activity of individual, age, and pre-existing illness.

(continues)

(Heat Emergencies, continued)

HEAT STROKE RESPONSE GUIDE

QUESTIONS	RESPONSES	ACTION TO TAKE	RATIONALE
Does the victim have red and hot skin, pupils dilated, rapid pulse, altered mental state? 　　　NO 　　　➡	YES ◊	Office calls 911 for caller. ◊ Have caller immediately lower body temperature by removing the victim from the sun, removing any heavy clothing, applying wet sheets, and fanning the patient. Continue cooling until body reaches 103°F. Give nothing by mouth. Monitor the patient.	Immediate action is necessary to avoid death. Body temperature must be reduced. Important to maintain reduced body temperature. Always call 911 because victim needs hospital care.
Consult physician.			Physician has final decision whether patient is seen.

Seizures

While few seizures require medical attention, they can be a frightening experience for the unaware. Office personnel need to understand that the caller will need a great deal of support. If the caller is unaware of a diagnosis of seizure activity, the EMS system will need to be called immediately. Useful information can be gathered from observers of the seizure activity, and the office should encourage these observations. The emergency procedure for tonic-clonic seizure activity will be covered here; for additional information see Chapter 11, page 155.

Tonic-Clonic seizures are characterized by:

1. The prodromal state—headaches and mood changes.
2. Aura—visual, olfactory, auditory sensation or motor activity in one area of the body.
3. Loss of consciousness.
4. Tonic phase—substandard contraction of all voluntary muscles: lasts 10–30 seconds.
5. Clonic phase—intermittent contractions and relaxation of skeletal muscle. Lasts from seconds to minutes. After muscle contractions cease, patient is cyanotic and unresponsive. Patient may become incontinent.
6. Postictal stage—patient may be drowsy or semi-conscious and may want to sleep for several hours.

Immediate medical attention is needed for the condition of status epilepticus—seizures that last over 5 minutes or are recurrent. This condition causes severe respiratory compromise and is life-threatening.

(continues)

SEIZURE RESPONSE GUIDE

QUESTIONS	RESPONSES	ACTION TO TAKE	RATIONALE
Is patient experiencing any of the following: • rigidity? • spastic moves? • clenching of the teeth? • loss of awareness of surroundings? NO ➡	YES ◊	• Instruct caller to protect head; move objects away from patient. • **DO NOT** restrain patient or force anything in patient's mouth. • Assure caller it is impossible to swallow the tongue. • Loosen any tight fitting clothing, belts, collars, etc. • Observe patient closely. Note the time seizure began and ended. Office should stay on the phone with the caller.	Patient needs to be protected during seizure activity.
Has there been fever present at any time? NO ➡			
Consult physician.			Physician has final decision whether patient is seen.

(Seizures, continued)

NOTE: If seizure lasts longer than 5 minutes or if seizures are recurrent, call EMS immediately. This condition is known as status epilepticus and is a medical emergency.
(Seizures are covered more fully in Chapter 11.)

Fever

Many things can affect the body's temperature. Viruses, bacteria, exposure to the sun, and hormones all affect the core body temperature. The average body temperature is 98.6°F, but it varies from individual to individual. It is a good idea for patients to take their temperatures when they are well, to establish a baseline. Most office calls concerning a fever are about children. This guide deals with children only.

FEVER RESPONSE GUIDE

QUESTIONS	RESPONSES	ACTION TO TAKE	RATIONALE
Is the child less than 3 months old? NO	YES ◊	Patient to come to office. ◊	Infants can dehydrate rapidly with an elevated body temperature.
Has there been a seizure or is breathing rapid? NO	YES ◊	Patient to come to office. ◊	Child needs to be evaluated.
Are there any other physical complaints? NO	YES ◊	Patient to come to office. ◊	Patient needs to be seen.
Has the fever lasted over 72 hours? NO	YES ◊	Patient to come to office. ◊	Temperatures that remain elevated require medical attention.
			It is impossible to evaluate the child over the phone.
Consult physician.			Physician has final decision whether patient is seen.

Animal Bites

The greatest concern with animal bites is rabies, carried by wild animals, especially skunks, foxes, bats, raccoons, and opossums. It is extremely rare in squirrels, chipmunks, rats, and field mice. Rabid animals act strangely, attack without provocation, and often foam at the mouth. While animal bites cause the most damage to tissue, human bites are more dangerous because of the chance of contamination when the skin is broken. Human bites are treated in the same manner as animal bites; however, due to the increased risk of infections, these patients should be seen.

ANIMAL BITE RESPONSE GUIDE

QUESTIONS	RESPONSES	ACTION TO TAKE	RATIONALE
Is the face involved? NO ➛	YES ◊	Patient to come to office ◊ immediately. Report all dog and cat bites to the health department.	There may be potential cosmetic disfigurement.
If bitten by a dog or cat, are immunizations of the animal current? Has the animal been confined? NO ➛	YES ◊	Patient to come to office. ◊	Patient will need to be evaluated by the physician. Have caller wash animal bite of any type thoroughly with soap and water. Bites should be cleaned ASAP.
Has the bite left a cut or puncture wound? NO ➛ Consult physician.	YES ◊	Patient to come to office. ◊	Puncture wounds require an updated tetanus shot. Physician has final decision whether patient is seen.

NOTE: If the animal is identified and there is no proof of immunization available, the animal must be confined for observation. It is best if the Animal Control Center is called to capture the animal.

Burns

Burns are classified as first, second, or third degree (Figures 3-6 and 3-7). First degree burns are usually sunburns; they are painful but seldom need medical attention. Second degree burns are painful, have blisters, and can cause significant fluid loss. Any second degree burn that involves an area bigger than a child's hand should be seen in the office. If the burn involves the face, hands, feet, or genitals, the burn should be seen by a physician. Third degree burns destroy all layers of the skin and extend into deeper tissue. Charring is present. The burn is often painless due to the destruction of nerve endings. All third degree burns should be seen by EMS or a physician. Each type of burn and its care will be presented.

FIRST DEGREE BURN RESPONSE GUIDE

QUESTIONS	RESPONSES	ACTION TO TAKE	RATIONALE
Is skin reddened without blisters? NO	YES ◊	Submerge in cool water ◊ 2–5 minutes.	Stops burning process.
Does area involve: • hands? • feet? • genitals? • face? NO	YES ◊	Patient to come to office. ◊	These are potential danger areas and require evaluation by the physician.
Is patient: • elderly? • very young? NO	YES ◊	Patient to come to office. ◊	These groups are very susceptible to burn complications.
Consult physician.			Physician has final decision whether patient is seen.

(continues)

(Burns, continued)

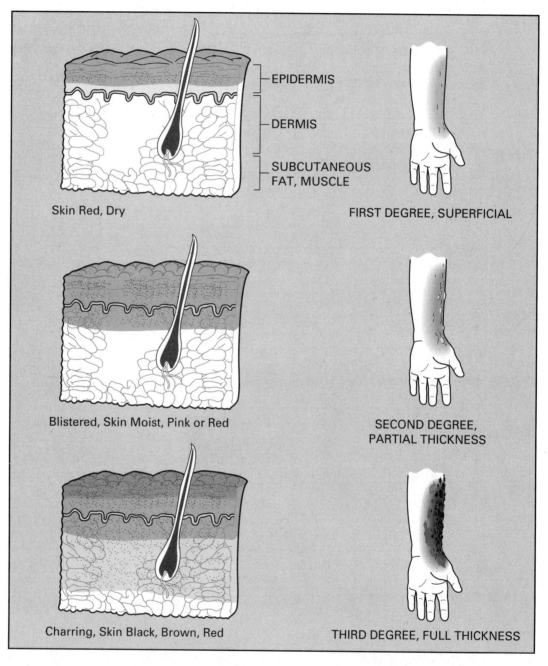

Skin Red, Dry

FIRST DEGREE, SUPERFICIAL

EPIDERMIS

DERMIS

SUBCUTANEOUS FAT, MUSCLE

Blistered, Skin Moist, Pink or Red

SECOND DEGREE, PARTIAL THICKNESS

Charring, Skin Black, Brown, Red

THIRD DEGREE, FULL THICKNESS

Figure 3-6   Burn depth classification. (Adapted from Eichelberger, Ball, Pratsch, and Runion, *Pediatric Emergencies: A Manual for Prehospital Care Providers*. © 1992. Adapted by permission of Prentice-Hall, Englewood Cliffs, New Jersey.)

(Burns, continued)

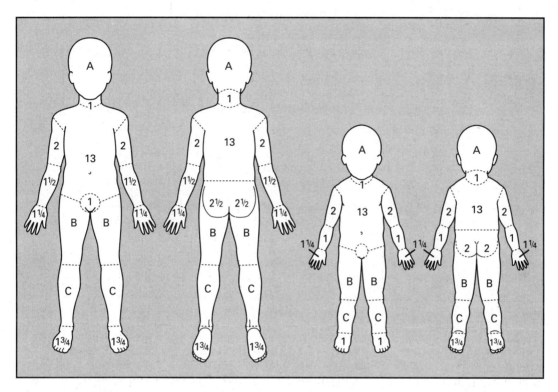

Figure 3-7 The extent of a child's burn is estimated using the Lund and Browder formula, which indicates relative percentages of areas affected. (Adapted from Artz and Moncrief, *The Treatment of Burns,* 2nd Edition, W. B. Saunders, 1969.)

(Burns, continued)

SECOND DEGREE BURN RESPONSE GUIDE

QUESTIONS	RESPONSES	ACTION TO TAKE	RATIONALE
Is skin reddened with blisters or splitting of the skin? NO ➡	YES ◊	Submerge in cool water ◊ 10–15 minutes if skin is intact. Use compresses if skin is broken. Do not break blisters. Do not use anesthetic creams or sprays.	Stops burning process. If blisters are broken, can allow infection in burn. Creams or spray may slow healing process and increase severity of a burn.
Does area involve: • hands? • feet? • genitals? • face? NO ➡	YES ◊	Patient to come to office. ◊	These are potentially dangerous areas and require medical attention.
Is the area involved larger than a child's hand? NO ➡	YES ◊	Patient to come to office. ◊	Burns of this size are very susceptible to complications.
Is patient experiencing trouble breathing? NO ➡	YES ◊	Patient to come to office. ◊	There may be swelling of the airways because of heat.
Consult physician.			Physician has final decision whether patient is seen.

(Burns, continued)

THIRD DEGREE BURN RESPONSE GUIDE

QUESTIONS	RESPONSES	ACTION TO TAKE	RATIONALE
Is skin gray, black, or charred appearing? Can muscle, fat, or bone be seen in wound? NO ⬦	YES ⟡	Call EMS immediately. ⟡ Do not apply cold; do not remove burnt clothing from burn area.	Life-threatening emergency that requires prompt attention.
Is patient experiencing: • pallor? • loss of consciousness? • shivering? NO ⬦	YES ⟡	Patient in shock: ⟡ • maintain body temp. • elevate feet if appropriate. • monitor breathing.	Need to control shock due to loss of fluid.
Consult physician.			Physician has final decision whether patient is seen.

Fractures

Any time there is a reasonable suspicion of a fracture, an X ray will be required. This guide is provided to identify instances where an X ray is recommended. Signs and symptoms of a fracture may include shock, pain, swelling, shortened or deformed limb, and bruising. Often, a fracture cannot be distinguished from a sprain or dislocation without an X ray (see Figure 3-8).

Callers in all cases should be instructed to apply ice to reduce swelling and inflammation. The joint above and below the bone should be immobilized. Magazines, cardboard, and rolled newspapers can be used for splints. Do not wrap tightly, as it will prevent adequate circulation. Time is not a factor unless there is profuse bleeding or injury to the nerves or blood vessels. Any injury still painful after 48 hours needs evaluation by the physician.

FRACTURE RESPONSE GUIDE

QUESTIONS	RESPONSES	ACTION TO TAKE	RATIONALE
Is the limb cold, blue, or numb? NO ⬇	YES ▷	Patient to come to ▷ office or go to ER.	Fractures can injure nerves and arteries.
Does area involve: • pelvic region? • thigh? NO ⬇	YES ▷	Patient to come to office ▷ or go to ER.	These fractures can result in internal bleeding and shock.
Is the limb unusable and/or nonweight-bearing? NO ⬇	YES ▷	Patient to come to office ▷ or go to ER.	If pain prevents the use of the limb, it may indicate a fracture.
Is there a great deal of bleeding and bruising in the area? Was the injury the result of a severe blow? NO ⬇	YES ▷	Patient to come to office ▷ or go to ER.	Needs to be evaluated.
Consult physician.			Physician has final decision whether patient is seen.

(Continues)

(Fractures, continued)

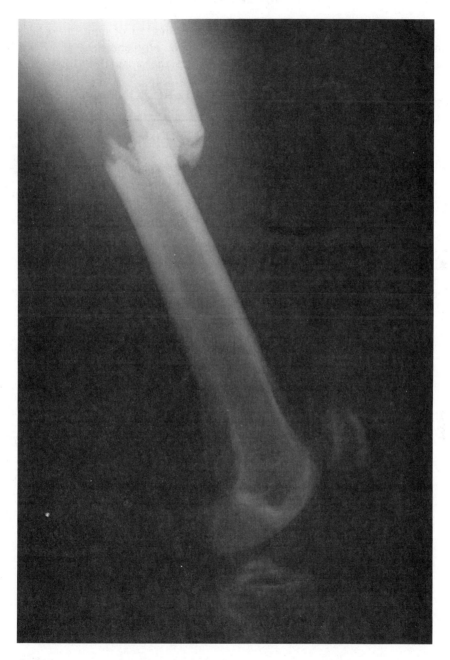

Figure 3-8 X ray showing a fractured femur. (From Burke, *Human Anatomy & Physiology in Health and Disease,* 3rd ed., © 1992, Delmar Publishers.)

Eye Pain/Foreign Body in Eye

All eye injuries should be taken seriously. Infection and loss of sight can result from a mismanaged situation involving an eye. Most minor problems with an eye will heal within 48 hours. If there is a complaint after 48 hours, the patient must see the physician.

EYE PAIN/FOREIGN BODY IN EYE RESPONSE GUIDE

QUESTIONS	RESPONSES	ACTION TO TAKE	RATIONALE
Are any of the following present? • visible foreign body • blood in the eye • feeling of irritation in the eye NO ➡	YES ◊	Patient to see physician ◊ immediately or call EMS.	Must be evaluated immediately.
Is there any problem with vision? NO ➡	YES ◊	Patient to come to office. ◊	Requires evaluation.
Is there eye pain? NO ➡	YES ◊	Patient to come to office. ◊	Requires evaluation.
Consult physician.			Physician has final decision whether patient is seen.

Pain

Pain is a symptom of a problem and needs to be investigated. Often medical personnel can obtain information about the pain that can give a clue as to the urgency of the problem. What is recommended for the pain will be determined by the response. Each office should discuss what action is to be taken.

PAIN RESPONSE GUIDE

QUESTIONS	RATIONALE
Severity of the pain? • dull • sharp • stabbing • crushing • knifing Is pain: • intermittent? • constant? • only at certain times? Changes in pain: • what makes it better? • what makes it worse? How long has the pain been present?	Learn as much about the pain as possible to determine if it is an emergency or not. The patient determines if there is an emergency. Pain is a symptom of something wrong and should never be ignored by medical personnel. Chest pain—activate EMS.

Chest Pain

Chest pain can be caused by a variety of problems, including ischemic disorders (lack of adequate oxygen to the heart), pleurisy, and stomach and gallbladder problems. Stress, indigestion, and anxiety can also cause or aggravate chest pains. It is important to remember that the individual and family members are usually very apprehensive about this type of pain and frequently deny cardiac involvement. Depending upon the reaction of the caller and the physician's preference, it might be best to activate the EMS immediately.

CHEST PAIN RESPONSE GUIDE

QUESTIONS	RESPONSES	ACTION TO TAKE	RATIONALE
Are any of these conditions present for the first time? • shortness of breath • pain that radiates to the neck, jaw, or arms • irregular or rapid pulse • sudden onset of pain NO	YES ◊	Call EMS. ◊	Sudden severe chest pain may indicate life-threatening situation.
Does the patient take nitroglycerin for chest pain? NO	YES ◊	Patient should take 1 ◊ tablet every 5 min. × 3. If pain continues, call EMS.	Patient may have been diagnosed with angina and prescribed nitroglycerin.
Are any of the following present? • fatigue • epistaxis • abdominal pain • nonproductive cough NO	YES ◊	Have patient come to ◊ office ASAP.	Other disorders produce chest pain in addition to other symptoms. Examples may be pneumonia, pericarditis, or indigestion.
Does the patient have a history of heart problems? NO Consult physician.	YES ◊	Patient to come to office ◊ or call EMS.	Patient may be experiencing another cardiac episode. Physician has final decision whether patient is seen.

Diabetic Coma

Diabetic coma is caused by increased blood sugar. Overindulgence of foods that contain or produce sugar, too little insulin, or decreased activity can contribute to the condition known as diabetic coma. The body, unable to convert the sugar into usable energy, breaks down fat stored in the body, and ketoacidosis occurs (acid-like substance in the bloodstream). If left untreated, diabetic acidosis causes unconsciousness and eventually death.

DIABETIC COMA RESPONSE GUIDE

QUESTIONS	RESPONSES	ACTION TO TAKE	RATIONALE
Is the patient experiencing: • thirst? • abdominal pain? • nausea? • vomiting? • slight fever? Is the patient's skin dry? Is there a sweetish smell to the breath? Do the eyeballs appear sunken and soft? NO	YES ◊	If patient is conscious, ◊ give fluids (water) and transport immediately. If patient is unconscious, transport immediately.	Life-threatening emergency that requires prompt attention.
Is the pulse rapid? Is the patient complaining of headache, restlessness, or dim vision? NO Consult physician.	YES ◊	See above. ◊	There are many different symptoms to this situation. Physician has final decision whether patient is seen.

Diabetic coma is covered more fully in Chapter 11.

Insulin Shock

Insulin shock occurs because of too much insulin, not enough food, increased exercise, and waiting too long to eat. Patients will need immediate medical care. If the caller is unsure as to why the symptoms are occurring, the conscious victim should be given sugar or sugar-containing beverages.

INSULIN SHOCK RESPONSE GUIDE

QUESTIONS	RESPONSES	ACTION TO TAKE	RATIONALE
Is patient known diabetic? Is patient experiencing: • headache? • cold sweat? • poor coordination? • staggering gait? • slurred speech? • emotional changes? • numbness or tingling? NO ↧	YES ◊	Give conscious ◊ victim sugar or sugar-containing beverage. Monitor patient reaction. Keep caller on the phone. If victim is ◊ unconscious, contact EMS.	Need to boost sugar level ASAP. Do not give anything by mouth to an unconscious victim, as aspiration may occur.
What symptoms are seen by caller? NO ↧ Consult physician	Responses will vary. ◊	Patient to come to ◊ office/contact EMS. Further investigation necessary.	Hard to determine over phone. Physician has final decision whether patient is seen.

Insulin shock is covered more fully in Chapter 11.

Asthma

Asthma can be divided into extrinsic and intrinsic types. Asthmatics, regardless of the cause or type, suffer from hyperirritable airways. The result is oversensitivity to a substance, causing an airway obstruction due to bronchospasm, swelling of mucous membranes, and plugging of the bronchi by thick secretions. A severe prolonged asthmatic attack is an immediate medical emergency, known as status asthmaticus. The victim becomes exhausted and dehydrated due to the great difficulty of attempting to move air into the lungs.

ASTHMA RESPONSE GUIDE

QUESTIONS	RESPONSES	ACTION TO TAKE	RATIONALE
Is wheezing present? NO ➡	YES ◊	Come to office. ◊	Requires evaluation.
Does patient have: • dry skin? • dull eyes? • sunken eyeballs? • poor skin turgor? (If skin is gently pinched, it does not return to original shape quickly.) NO ➡	YES ◊	Transport to nearest ◊ medical facility.	Patient is showing classic symptoms of dehydration and needs to be evaluated for the cause.
Is patient experiencing unproductive cough, rapid respiration, or shortness of breath? NO ➡	YES ◊	Transport to the office. ◊	Requires evaluation.
Consult physician.			Physician has final decision whether patient is seen.

Asthma is covered more fully in Chapter 6.

Summary

Because the telephone is a basic link between the office and patients, office staff need a quick and easy reference system approved by the physician. Developing a telephone emergency response guideline for the modern health office avoids the legal pitfalls of giving advice over the telephone; it reduces the chances of having wrong or misleading information given to patients, and it lessens the helplessness that office staff feel when dealing with emergencies over the telephone. Offices should always call the patient back to assure a satisfactory progress, at the same time allowing follow-up documentation, and working to improve the relationship between the office staff and the patient.

Review Questions

1. Explain the importance of the telephone in an emergency situation.

2. What type of problems can arise if the office personnel put a patient on hold without expressed permission?

3. Why is it important to keep a calm, reassuring, even tone of voice on the telephone to an anxious patient or caller?

4. List a potential complication to using a stock phrase such as, "Everything will be OK."

5. Explain the importance of a procedural sheet for dealing with telephone emergencies.

6. What changes might be made on the telephone procedural sheets?

7. Why should the physician be consulted if the appropriate questions do not provide sufficient information for the office staff?

8. Why should the office personnel spend the time with patients on the phone? Why not just make an appointment?

9. A call comes in for a physician who will not be in the office. What are the appropriate steps the office personnel should take?

CHAPTER 4

Documentation

Objectives

After completing this chapter the learner should be able to:

1. List six purposes of documentation.
2. Identify and describe the two major methods of documentation.
3. Define the difference between subjective and objective charting.
4. List the four most common recordkeeping errors.
5. Follow appropriate guidelines for documentation.
6. Accurately record the emergency on an incident report.

Introduction

Documentation is the written picture of an event. It is essential to communicate current information in order to facilitate and verify a standard of care. Accurate descriptive terms can convey a wealth of information. Documentation serves a variety of important purposes including:

    1. Quality of care. Accurate documentation describes the patient's medical emergencies. It verifies that quality care was provided to the patient.

2. Coordination of care. To provide patient with the best possible care, it is important that medical team members have complete information on what was done for the patient.

3. Accurate medical records. Record pertinent patient information.

4. Insurance reimbursement. Insurance companies need a written description of the care in order to determine patient reimbursement.

5. Create a legal record. Patient records are legal documents that can be subpoenaed into court if problems arise from care. Therefore, be able to document justification for any emergency care provided.

6. Allow for evaluation of staff personnel. Staff should meet after an emergency situation and critique each individual's emergency skills.

Charting Methods

Charting can be organized in one of two basic methods: source-oriented and problem-oriented. Each physician will choose which method best fits the needs of the office.

Source-oriented Method

Source-oriented narrative form is seldom used in the office situation, but is used in large health care facilities around the country. This method requires each member of the health care team to record information in a separate section of the patient's file: lab personnel in one area, nurses in another, doctors in yet another. Communication among health care team members is difficult with separate sheets of documentation, so color-coded sheets of paper are used. Everything is in chronological order without identifying the topic of documentation. The problem-oriented method below solves these problems.

Problem-oriented Method

A common methodology used in the medical office is the problem-oriented medical record. There are four basic components to this type of documentation: compilation of baseline information, a problem list, an initial plan for each designated problem, and progress notes.

Baseline information focuses on the patient's present complaints and illnesses. Included are social and emotional information, medical status, medical history, results from the initial physical examination, and diagnostic test results. The office can use these results to evaluate the patient on subsequent visits.

The **problem list** includes what brought the patient to the office (often recorded by the health care professional), problems identified by the physician after further discussion with the patient, and information about any problems with tests that had been run. The problem list can serve as an indicator for the office as to possible complications, treatment, and education the patient will require.

The **initial treatment** is established by the physician after a diagnosis is made or while further testing is being done. Plans will include collecting further data, treatment (which may include medication), therapy, and/or surgical interventions. The patient education plan should be included in the documentation; it should include what needs to be taught and who is to conduct the patient education. Diabetic education is directed toward insulin injections and/or dietary changes. The health care members will use this portion of the chart to obtain information regarding the plans of the physician for the patient's treatment.

The **progress notes** allow the office personnel to track changes in a patient's condition. The progress notes are also used to document the Subjective, Objective, Assessment, and Plan, referred to as SOAP.

The advantages of this method are improved communication between the physician and office staff, quick access to the patient's problems, and well-organized information. A disadvantage is the repetition that occurs—the problem list will repeat what is done in the SOAP format.

Most offices will use an abbreviated form of this method. It is important that the office staff be totally familiar with the methodology used and that there is a standardized format used for every patient chart.

Subjective and Objective Charting

When charting, the office staff will need to differentiate between what the patient says and what the health care professional notices.

Subjective Charting

Subjective charting is writing down what the patient says. Often the allied health professional must "sift" through a dialogue by the patient in order to reduce the complaint to a maximum of three sentences or less. Physicians require two things from the charting of their staff: accuracy and brevity. Using standard charting abbreviation will facilitate both elements.

When repeating exactly what the patient has said, enclose it in quotation marks. For example, the patient states, "My head hurts." Health care professionals should be careful never to make a diagnosis or interpret what the patient is saying. If the patient claims to have a condition, the allied health professional should ask why the patient believes it is that particular condition and only chart the symptoms as the patient relates them. The physician is the only one who can make a diagnosis.

Objective Charting

Objective charting is documenting what the medical assistants or allied health professionals observe on their own. Some examples would be: pallor, diaphoresis, flushed face, trembling, vital signs, and so on. Every effort should be made to use the correct medical terminology. Any documentation is subject to subpoena in a court of law; it should be an accurate and descriptive picture of the patient's care.

Common Recordkeeping Errors

The four most common recordkeeping errors in the medical office are:

1. Charting subjective information as a statement. This appears in the chart as if the staff has made a diagnosis.
2. Mistakes in the chart, such as date, wrong patient's chart, and so on. The medical personnel should draw one line through the mistake and then date and initial the error. Nursing/medical schools in this area teach **never** to write "error"—just to line through and initial. In some areas, the health professionals may be requested to write "error" above with their initials and the corrections.
3. Documenting before the fact. Never write a procedure down as completed until it is. Often the personnel will attempt to simplify the steps to a procedure by charting it before it takes place. Because the chart is a legal document, never chart any procedure, such as an injection, unless it has been done. If the physician has written the order, then after the procedure is completed, the office personnel should initial the order to indicate it has been completed.
4. Failure to document. Always document immediately after the situation has been resolved. If it is an emergency situation, one member of the staff should document during the emergency care. If this is not possible, the charting should be done immediately following the emergency to ensure accuracy and completeness.

General Guidelines

In order to ensure that accurate information is compiled in the patient's chart, the following guidelines should be followed:

1. Record only the facts. Never use the patient's chart to record opinions or guesses of the medical personnel. An unfactual remark written in the chart can destroy the credibility of the entire file.

2. Always write everything down. If it is not written down, it didn't happen. When in doubt, document everything.

3. Document objectively. Document what is seen, done, and heard. If charting a patient's statement, use the exact wording and put in quotation marks. (Only record facts, not opinions or guesses.)

4. Reduce charting to the least number of words while retaining accuracy. Avoid charting unnecessary or unrelated information.

5. Initial entries as they are made. Records are a permanent, legal document. Use black ink because it photocopies well.

6. Only use standard abbreviations. A list from the local hospital of accepted abbreviations will help.

7. Spell correctly. If unsure of a spelling, look it up. Use medical terminology to avoid misunderstanding and to convey professional behavior.

8. Write legibly. Illegible writing can hinder communication and lead to errors in patient care. In litigation, it creates an unfavorable impression and can be interpreted as negligence.

9. Correct errors promptly, using the correct format.

10. Write on every line. Never leave blank lines on the chart. Draw a line through empty spaces, thus preventing others from inserting information.

11. Always identify the patient. Be sure the patient's name, ID number, and allergies (in large red letters) appear on each page of the file.

Emergency Recordkeeping

Following each emergency, a chronological descriptive picture of the event must be entered into the patient's chart. As shown in Figure 4-1, documentation should include:

Emergency Documentation Form

Patient Name _____   Date of Birth _____

Sex _____

Date _____

Time _____

V.S.

    Pulse _____   Resp _____

Time _____ Rate   Time _____ Rate _____

B/P   Temperature

Time _____ Rate   Time _____ Rate _____

Patient's Complaints

Signs and Symptoms

Current Meds

Actions Taken

Name of physician and individuals involved in providing care

Referrals—Physician/Facility

Figure 4-1.   Emergency documentation form.

- Description of patient before, during, and after the emergency.
- Vital signs.
- Any medication given, including name, strength, route, dosage given, and who administered it.
- If oxygen was administered, how it was given, flow rate, and percentage.
- If any other emergency techniques were administered, they should be described. Include the time each action was taken.
- All office personnel should initial the documentation, and the physician should sign off on it.

Documentation not only provides a written picture of patient care, but serves as a legal document in case there are questions as to what was done to and for the patient. A member of the health care team should be made responsible for documenting during the emergency. If this is not possible, every effort should be made to document immediately following the emergency to ensure an accurate depiction of the event.

Summary

Accurate and complete documentation is essential to protect the individuals—physicians, office personnel, and patients—from the ethical and legal pitfalls of dealing with an emergency, and it also provides for quality follow-up care.

Review Questions

1. Define the following terms as they relate to documentation:
   a. Quality of care.
   b. Coordination of care.
   c. Insurance reimbursement.
   d. Legal record.
2. Why is communication among health care members a problem when using the source-oriented narrative?
3. Define baseline information and how its use can improve patient care in a medical office.
4. How does a patient's record give clues as to what education is required for the patient?

5. The patient complains of headache, nausea, and vomiting. Which of these are subjective findings and which are objective findings? Explain why.

6. List the four most common recordkeeping errors and a suggestion on how to avoid each one.

7. Why is the statement, "If it's not charted, it didn't happen," true?

8. List one thing that can cause an unfavorable impression in litigation when documenting in a patient's chart.

9. Chart the significant information:

Sam Smith comes into the office complaining of headache, right arm pain, and a feeling of suffocation. He says that an elephant is sitting on his chest. His right leg is mottled and blue. Pulse is 130 and weak, breathing is 35, blood pressure is 180/60. His wife has driven him to the office after he got off work at 4:30 p.m. His two daughters are at home with their grandmother, who suffered a myocardial infarction last year, but gets around well on her own. His wife says all the stress and Sam's anger have caused her to feel nauseated.

CHAPTER 5

Applications and Techniques of Psychological First Aid

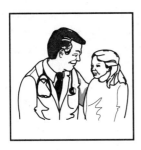

Objectives

After completing this chapter the learner should be able to:

1. Recognize psychological distress.
2. Select the appropriate method of dealing with an individual's distress.
3. Identify legal and ethical issues surrounding patient care in a crisis situation.
4. Assess the individual's psychological state and apply the appropriate communication techniques.
5. Explain when open-ended questions are appropriate in an emergency situation.
6. Explain when closed questions are appropriate in emergency situations.

Introduction

Any emergency situation has the potential for becoming unmanageable due to the psychological factors involved. Every individual will respond differently in a crisis situation; the medical professional needs to be prepared to deal with a variety of unexpected behaviors from victims, family members, and bystanders.

In any crisis, the situation will be impacted by a number of variables. First, who is the victim? If the person in psychological distress is the victim, the situation will be handled differently from one in which the individual in psychological distress is a family member or a bystander.

Each individual has personal resources, internal strengths that they may have developed in order to cope with unsettling circumstances. These resources typically mean that some people are better equipped to cope with distress than others.

Another variable revolves around the resources that are available during the time of psychological distress. A professional, short-term support system needs to be functioning within the medical setting.

Basic Skills for Communication

The basic skills that the professional will need are the ability to:

- Observe.
- Verbally communicate.
- Use and interpret nonverbal communication.
- Listen.

Each of these skills helps to provide a supportive, helpful environment for patients and families.

The goal of psychological first aid is to strengthen or restore the ability of the individual to cope with the immediate situation. It is not possible to describe every potential circumstance. The medical professional will need to apply basic skills to a given situation and use considered adaptation when necessary.

Patients experiencing normal psychological distress need to have medical personnel support. (Techniques used to convey this support are discussed later in the chapter.) Patients experiencing increasing difficulties with the emergency situation will require a larger amount of the office personnel's time and energy. Patients who are affected severely should never be left alone. Close attention helps to lessen their sense of detachment, allowing the staff to observe them and implement any measures needed to protect the patient and the staff from harm.

Skills for Dealing with Patients and Family in the Office

The following seven hints will be helpful for dealing with patients and family:

1. Know the power of touch.
2. Listen.
3. Validate the person's emotions.
4. Do not feel you need to give the right answer.
5. Do not be afraid of tears—the patient's or your own.
6. Remember that hearing is the last sense to go.
7. Be yourself.

Observation

In order to assist these patients, the medical professional must be able to identify those individuals who are experiencing psychological distress. Depending upon situational circumstances and individual responses, signs of distress will be expressed in a variety of ways. However, there are common physical signs that everyone experiences after an emergency. They include shakiness, heavy breathing, perspiration, rapid breathing, tachycardia, dilated pupils, faintness, and nausea. Normally, these reactions will subside after a short period of time. For some individuals these physical reactions can increase and create a type of psychological paralysis that causes the patient to become incapacitated. Some patients will experience difficulty in concentrating, may have selective inattention, and may ask questions repetitively. In some cases, patients appear dazed and confused, unaware of what is going on around them. It is important for the medical personnel to observe patients for these signs and symptoms and be prepared to deal with a wide range of behavior. Always be alert for signs that indicate patients are gaining their composure, not losing it.

Verbal Communication

Patients who are experiencing distress will often benefit from the presence of another human being. The comfort of knowing that one does not have to deal with a difficult situation alone is immeasurable. Verbal communication is one method of establishing this therapeutic relationship. It is vital that the office personnel verbalize a supportive, calm, and caring attitude.

First, the office personnel should introduce themselves. Do not assume that patients always know the names of individuals in the office. Giving a name will help to establish office personnel as human beings the patient can relate to. If the patient is unfamiliar with the office, make the introductions bilateral. "Hello. My name is Jane Williams. I'm Dr. Smith's medical assistant. Your name is Judy Mansfield?" This will often allow the medical personnel to assess the orientation of the patient and give a clue as to what the patient prefers to be called, such as "Judy" instead of "Mrs. Mansfield."

The office personnel should be aware of their position in relationship to the patient. When beginning communication, the team member needs to be at eye level and in front of the patient. Patients may have difficulty relating to someone who towers over them. Also, some patients may be hearing-impaired and will need to lip-read.

Verbalization of an understanding of their feelings is also an important part of establishing a supportive relationship. "I understand how upsetting this must be," can convey support and caring to the patient. The voice itself should be pitched low to produce a calming effect; for those individuals with hearing disabilities, the tone is easier to hear.

Be sure that an explanation of what is happening, what is being done, and what is going to happen next is given to the distressed patient. Patients who are told why a procedure is being done are more likely to comply with and help office personnel. It will create a working relationship for all involved in the emergency situation. Even patients who are unconscious should be given explanations as to their treatment, as there is substantial evidence that individuals who are unconscious or in a coma can hear these explanations. It is important to remember that coma patients may recall what was said during their treatment. The health care worker should be careful not to say anything that could cause problems at a future date.

Tell patients that it is appropriate to express their feelings. People do not know how they should behave in an emergency situation. The office personnel must assess patients' reactions. If they pose no threat to staff or themselves, verbalize acceptance of this behavior: "It's OK to cry. I know it must hurt." Often this conveys to patients that it is OK to react to the situation, helping to build trust and rapport between the personnel involved and the patients.

Reassurance should be given often and repeatedly. It is vital that the reassurance given does not include a promise of "Everything will be fine." Expressions like "I'm here with you" or "The doctor will be here soon" are all acceptable phrases of reassurance. Inappropriate phrases such as "You'll be fine" or "There's no pain involved" can lead to ethical and legal problems. Telling a patient everything will be OK can be seen as a guarantee from the doctor. Everything is not OK for all patients, and the phrase could result in legal action by the patients and/or their family members. Telling a patient that a procedure will not hurt can damage the level of trust that the office personnel has worked to establish.

It should be remembered that words mean little if the action of personnel contradict them. Nonverbal techniques should be employed to strengthen the therapeutic relationship established through verbal communication.

Nonverbal Communication

The use of the body to convey meaning is very much a part of our culture. Different countries have various gestures to express different things, but all humans, regardless of the language spoken, use this type of communication. Basic body language is used to make speech more effective.

In most cases, body language provides an emphasis to the spoken word. However, body language can contradict a spoken message. In these instances, studies have shown that body language is trusted over what the professional actually says. For example, an individual was asked to say something pleasant in a hostile tone, and the people in the study, disregarding the words spoken, judged the individual's attitude as hostile. Being sure that body language matches the words will help the office staff to reassure patients more effectively. The secret lies in the ability to use appropriate cues with the correct amount of intensity and to always remain responsive to the patient.

Eye Contact

It has been said that the eyes are the windows of the soul. Perhaps that is why people are very leery about how often they look into someone else's eyes. However, the eyes do show a large variety of emotions and can be used quite successfully to gauge a person's mood or feelings. Looking at the eyes can tell the medical personnel a lot about how a person is feeling, regardless of what the mouth is saying.

Eye contact is also an excellent vehicle to express honest emotions. As the medical office personnel work to establish a rapport with the patient, the use of eye contact should not be overlooked. Most people are more willing to trust someone who will make eye contact than someone who avoids it.

It is necessary to practice the use of eye contact in order to achieve a degree of proficiency. Many people respond unconsciously to eye signals every day. By being aware of these (unconscious) mood signals, the office personnel can learn to assess more reliably the moods of the patient and family members.

Facial Expression

There are six basic emotions that can be recognized by facial expression: happiness, sadness, anger, disgust, surprise, and fear. Medical personnel may observe the patient's face for acceptance and comprehension of the situation. Certain facial expressions may denote the patient's need for further explanation.

On the reverse side, the office staff need to make sure that they are aware of their own facial expressions. Avoid overuse of facial expressions as these can be misinterpreted. For example, a blank face may be seen as a show of hostility or a lack of interest by the patient. Expressions that are badly timed, or that appear and fade quickly, can make the staff appear insincere. The face should match the feelings verbally expressed.

Interaction Distances

The physical distance maintained between patient and staff can affect how we use eye contact, touch, and orientation. Patients may react defensively if they feel crowded or feel that the medical personnel are forcing an intimacy that is not desired. Conversely, too much distance may imply that the staff are unfriendly and cold.

Distance can help to regulate interaction, especially when the medical personnel face the patient. The staff must judge the reaction of the patient to the distance and adjust accordingly. When the need for touching is indicated, office personnel or staff should maintain a professional detachment to reduce the potential for embarrassment. Minimizing touch allows the patient to maintain a comfortable personal space.

Posture

Slumped shoulders, bowed head, and folded arms may give an impression of disinterest, while a straight, erect head and open arms convey an attentive and caring posture.

Touch

Touching the patient/family briefly on the shoulder or arm conveys warmth, support, and caring. Remember the power of touch in an emergency situation.

Voice

The voice should be pitched at a moderate volume with varied pitch and varied pace.

Listening

Hearing and listening are not the same thing. People hear a lot of different sounds during the course of the day. Rarely, however, do they listen to those same sounds. The same observation can be made about conversation. How often has a conversation taken place that was only heard? Conscious effort is needed to listen to a patient. Some guidelines to become a good listener include use of supportive responses of understanding such as nods of the head, vocal feedback, eye contact, facial expressions, and appropriate body language.

It is important to the successful establishment of rapport that the patients feel that the medical professionals are listening to them. By using the above guidelines, the rapport between the patient and office staff can be increased.

Interviewing

An important task for medical personnel is to gather a complete history of the illness or injury from the patient and/or family.

An interview that uses both verbal and nonverbal communication will be the most thorough. Specific information needs to be gathered. The best place to start is the chief complaint. What brought the patient to the office? From that point, the medical personnel can fill in the details by asking directed questions.

The interviewing process needs to be flexible and adaptable to the individual situation. Appropriate questions, rather than a set of preselected questions, are the key to an interview that completes the picture of the emergency.

While in the beginning stages of the interview, most health professionals do rely on certain questions to ask. The ability to adapt these questions to the circumstances is an art form and needs constant revision and practice. However, there are certain rules that will help to develop the most effective interview process possible. First, always be sure that the question asked is in terminology that can be easily understood by the patient and family. As health care professionals learn new medical terms, there is a tendency to use this language, which can create confusion for lay people. Often the patient will have no idea what is being asked. Always try to phrase the question so that the patient can understand. For example:

Health Care Professional

"When did the trauma occur?"

Patient

"What do you mean, trauma?"

Health Care Professional

"The injury."

Patient

"Oh, I didn't understand."

Jargon

The use of jargon should also be avoided. Each culture has its own jargon and speech pattern that can create a communication barrier for patients and staff alike. If you are unsure as to the meaning of jargon, ask the patient to rephrase the statement. A humorous example of this is:

Health Care Professional

> "Hello, this is Clinic A."

Patient (male)

> "I need a check. I've been burned."

Health Care Professional

> "This clinic only deals with sexually transmitted diseases and pregnancy. For medical care for a burn, you will have to call your family doctor."

Patient

> "No. I mean I've been burned as in I've been with a gal that says she has the clap."

Health Care Professional

> "You mean gonorrhea?"

Patient

> "Yeah."

Open-ended or Closed Questions

The type of questions asked should be determined by how fast you need answers to provide the appropriate treatment. For example, a patient who is bleeding needs immediate treatment. Information can be gathered after care. Some patients will want to explain their whole life history, so questions will need to be very specific for sorting through all the information you receive.

The questions need to provide answers in the shortest and most effective way. Often health care professionals feel a time pressure in dealing with emergencies.

Questions can be closed or open-ended. If there is sufficient time or the patient keeps drifting off the point, ask open-ended questions. Open-ended questions require an exact response in the patient's own words:

- What were you doing at the time of the accident?
- What area(s) of your body hurt?

Closed questions require either a yes or no answer such as, "Can you feel your toes?"

Never ask questions that can be interpreted as accusatory. An example would be, "Why didn't you bring them to the office immediately following the accident?" These questions can cause hostility and impede the interview process. Carefully word your questions to project a positive professional attitude.

Common Barriers

Two common barriers to the interview are assumptions and sensory overload. Never assume what the history is. Allow the patient the opportunity to explain what occurred. The medical personnel must judge the honesty of the story but should never assume the answers.

Assumptions Often assumptions will cause wasted time in pursuing a line of questioning that is not indicated. One example would be an injury caused by a fall. Even though the patient appears intoxicated, the problem could be diabetes, head injury, or plain confusion.

Sensory Overload This is a particular problem with family members of the patient. Often seeing a loved one in pain or hurt can overwhelm the individual, and the ability to cope is diminished. Move the family member to a quiet place close to the patient but not in full sight. Allow the family member to readjust to the situation.

Summary

Any situation has the potential for becoming unmanageable, and the health care professional must be familiar with a variety of communication techniques in order to assess the situation, choose the best course of action, and tactfully take control to ensure as safe an environment as possible for all concerned. The professional should recognize that how a situation is approached can serve to put at ease an individual experiencing distress.

Communication techniques can be either verbal or nonverbal and include the art of listening. The health care professional will need to cultivate these skills to be effective in dealing with patients and others.

It is possible for a patient or family member to panic in an emergency and be unaware of actions that may cause additional injury to themselves or others. In a crisis situation, some individuals become a safety hazard because they are overwhelmed and find it difficult, if not impossible, to respond appropriately.

Our culture is comprised of a diverse population. Every individual has specific techniques for dealing with health emergencies. Based on past experience, cultural differences, and accurate or inaccurate knowledge, it is common for an untrained bystander to provide inappropriate care.

Potentially hazardous situations could include the behavior of individuals who have been accustomed to home remedy use. They may not fully understand the purpose of the medical environment and may impede medical care by becoming distraught or combative. The medical personnel will need to handle this type of situation in a calm, assertive manner to protect not only the patient, but also the bystander and other medical professionals.

Review Questions

1. Define the following types of communication and give an example of each:
   - Observation.
   - Verbal.
   - Nonverbal.
   - Listening.

2. Explain why nonverbal communication is so essential in finding out vital information.

3. List two common barriers to communication and how they can be overcome.

4. Develop an interview for the following patient, using the techniques outlined in this chapter:
   The patient is a 58-year-old male who has had difficulty working at his regular pace. He comes into the office: pulse 150, respiration rate of 23, blood pressure 190/100, diaphoretic, pale, gasping for air, complaining of numbness and tingling in the right arm. He denies having any history of heart problems and denies that it could be the problem now.

5. Explain how information in this chapter will help you in performing a patient assessment.

CHAPTER 6

Respiratory Emergencies

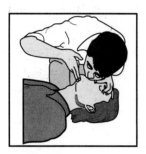

Objectives

After completing this chapter the learner should be able to:

1. Describe the functions of the respiratory system.

2. Identify the signs of respiratory distress.

3. Describe how to do patient assessment for respiratory distress.

4. Identify and list the steps and the appropriate procedure necessary to perform rescue breathing.

5. Identify the steps necessary to assist a person with an obstructed airway.

6. Identify the criteria necessary for choosing the appropriate airway for the patient.

7. Describe the procedure necessary for selecting the correct airway size for the patient.

8. List the proper steps for inserting both an oropharyngeal and a nasopharyngeal airway.

9. List the appropriate precautions to take when administering oxygen.

10. Describe the four different oxygen systems and the necessary criteria for their selection.

11. Define hyperventilation and the correct emergency treatment.

12. Define and explain the general guidelines for treating COPD.
13. Define emphysema and list the signs and symptoms.
14. Define chronic bronchitis and list the signs and symptoms.
15. List the treatment for bronchitis patients in distress.
16. Define asthma and list the signs and symptoms.
17. List the treatment for an acute asthma attack.
18. Define status asthmaticus.
19. Define pneumonia and list the signs and symptoms.
20. List the emergency care for a patient with pneumonia.

Introduction

Oxygen intake is essential for maintaining the body's functions. In emergency situations, the health care professional assessing an emergency patient should immediately make sure the patient is breathing and, if necessary, establish an open airway to facilitate breathing. Without the process of breathing and oxygen exchange, all other systems will cease to function, and the individual will die.

Anatomical Overview

The act of breathing is called respiration. As the individual breathes in (inspiration), oxygen is delivered to the lungs. The respiratory system is comprised of tube-like air passageways that have mucous-covered muscular lining. Air enters the nasal cavity, where it is warmed and filtered by mucous membrane and cilia, and then passes through the pharynx to the trachea. The larynx, which is also called the voice box, is located at the beginning of the trachea. As the cartilage-ringed trachea descends, it branches out to the bronchi, then continues to branch, progressively becoming smaller, much like an upside-down tree. The smallest branches, called bronchioles, end in the lungs as small air sacs called the alveoli (see Figure 6-1).

The thin-walled alveoli sacs are surrounded by blood capillaries. Oxygen that is inspired, or inhaled, diffuses from the alveoli into the blood capillaries. Carbon dioxide, a waste product of cellular metabolism, diffuses from the blood capillaries into the alveoli to be expired, or exhaled. The air is inhaled and exhaled by the contraction and relaxation of the diaphragm and chest muscles (see Figure 6-2).

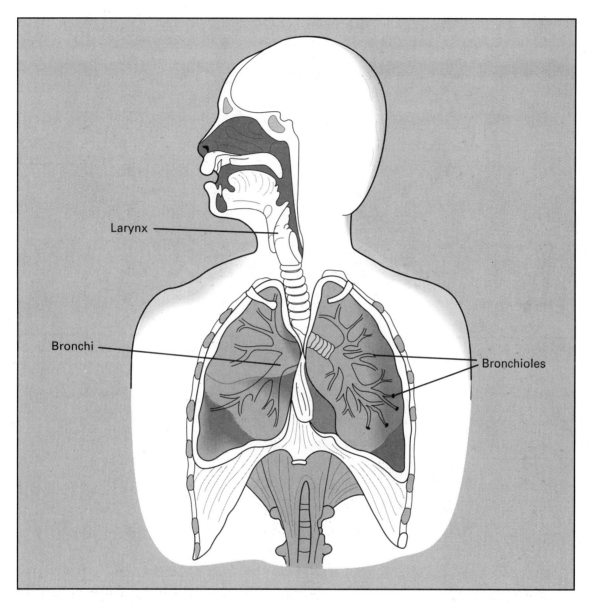

Figure 6-1 Respiratory system.

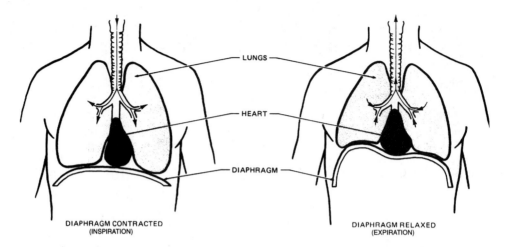

Figure 6-2   The action of the diaphragm muscle (Adapted from Krebs and Wise. *Medical Assisting, Clinical Competencies*, © 1994, Delmar Publishers.)

Respiratory Distress

There are degrees of respiratory distress that range from pulmonary insufficiency to pulmonary arrest. The signs and symptoms of distress are described in Table 6-1.

Table 6-1   Signs and Symptoms of Distress

Failure of the chest to rise and fall (in pediatric patients, failure of the abdomen to rise and fall).

Kussmaul—very rapid, deep respiration that resembles a sighing sound, which precedes a diabetic coma.

Bradypnea—abnormally slow breathing.

Noisy breathing (stertorous respiration)—snoring, gurgling, wheezing, etc.

Stridor—loud harsh breathing.

Depression of the skin that appears in the supraclavicular, intercostal, and substernal spaces.

Cyanosis—first observed in the fingernail beds and mucous membranes of the mouth.

Tachypnea—excessive, rapid breathing.

Progressive restlessness, anxiety, and confusion.

Movement of the Adam's apple in an upward motion on inhalation.

Medical personnel should be able to recognize these signs and symptoms in order to respond appropriately to the situation. Any of these presenting symptoms can lead to respiratory arrest; the medical professional will need to assess the situation and quickly implement proper emergency procedures. Respiratory difficulty can become a life-or-death situation.

While some situations may call for the use of breathing devices, medical personnel should not hesitate to begin patient assessment even though the equipment is not immediately at hand. At the first sign of an emergency, notify the physician of the situation and/or call 911.

Rescue Breathing

To begin patient assessment for an unconscious individual:

A. Establish unresponsiveness. Tap or gently shake the patient. Be sure to do both actions as some patients may be hard of hearing or deaf.

B. Look, listen, feel. Lean over the patient with the rescuer's face directed towards the patient's feet.

   1. Look to see if the chest is moving.
   2. Listen for air leaving the lungs.
   3. Feel for breath.

C. If the patient is not breathing, position properly. Position the patient on a flat, firm surface with the head even or slightly lower than the heart. The patient should be in a supine position. If the patient is on the abdomen or side, log roll the patient onto the back. Be careful to roll the body as a unit if there are suspected spinal injuries.

D. Airway:

   1. Tilt the head back by placing the hand on the patient's forehead and pushing back.
   2. Lift the chin by placing two fingers on the bony part of the chin and lifting.
   3. This technique opens the airway and breathing should be rechecked. The tongue is the most common cause of airway obstruction; this method causes the tongue to fall back out of the way.
   4. If a spinal injury is suspected, use the modified jaw thrust method.

E. Look, listen, feel, for 5 seconds.

F. If breathing is absent:

   1. Keep head tilted back; pinch the nose closed.

2. Use double end mouthpiece.

3. Give 2 slow breaths.

    a. Each breath should last 1 1/2 seconds.

    b. The patient's chest should rise.

    c. Lift your mouth from the mouthpiece between breaths.

G. Pulse:

1. Check for the pulse at the carotid artery.

2. Find the Adam's apple. Slide fingers down into the groove of the neck that is closest to you.

3. Check the pulse for 5–10 seconds. If there is a pulse—

H. Start rescue breathing.

1. Maintain head/chin tilt; pinch nose closed.

2. Give one slow breath every 5 seconds.

3. The patient's chest should rise.

4. Lift your mouth from the mouthpiece between breaths.

5. Continue giving breaths in this manner for approximately 1 minute, or 12 breaths (for an adult).

I. Recheck the pulse and breathing.

1. If a pulse and breathing are present:

    a. Stay with the patient.

    b. Keep the airway open.

    c. Monitor breathing.

2. If a pulse is present, but the patient is not breathing, continue with rescue breathing.

3. If a pulse and breathing are both absent, begin CPR.

Infant and child techniques differ slightly from those techniques used for an adult. The child's or infant's head is not tilted back as far as the adult's. A good rule to remember is "the smaller the individual, the less the head is tilted" (see Table 6-2 for the infant/child/adult comparison).

Airway Obstruction

Airway obstruction is the most common cause of respiratory emergencies. An obstructed airway can cause apnea, loss of consciousness, and death. There are 2 major causes of airway obstruction: (1) the tongue, or swollen tissues of the mouth and neck; and (2) a foreign object.

Table 6-2 Breathing Ratios for Adult, Child, and Infant

	Adult	**Child**	**Infant**
BREATHING	1 breath every 5 seconds	1 breath every 3 seconds	1 breath every 3 seconds
PULSE	Check at carotid artery	Check at carotid artery	Check at brachial artery
AMOUNT OF AIR	Until chest rises	Less air than adult	Puff of air

*Remember that children's and infants' heads are not tilted back as far as an adult's.

Common Causes of Airway Obstruction/Foreign Object Obstruction

Common causes of airway obstruction/foreign object obstruction include:

- Trying to swallow poorly chewed food.
- Drinking alcohol before and during meals.
- Wearing dentures.
- Talking or laughing while eating.
- Running with food or objects in the mouth.

Obstruction from a foreign object can cause either a partial or complete blockage of the airway.

Partial Airway Obstruction

Individuals with partial obstruction can still move air in and out of the lungs. This air assists the patient in attempting to dislodge the object by coughing. Partial airway obstruction is characterized by:

- Wheezing.
- The victim will clutch at the throat with one or both hands.
- The victim will be apprehensive.

Emergency Treatment

- If the patient is coughing forcefully, do not interfere.
- Stay with the patient.
- Encourage the patient to continue coughing to clear the obstruction.

Complete Airway Obstruction

Partial airway obstruction can become a complete obstruction. A patient with a complete airway obstruction will not be able to talk, cough, or breathe. Office personnel need to act immediately to save the patient's life.

Emergency care differs slightly depending upon whether the patient is conscious or unconscious, and on the patient's age. In either case, abdominal thrusts will be used to force trapped air up into the throat to dislodge the foreign object and push it out.

Conscious Choking—Adult/Child

A. Ask "Are you choking?" The patient may grab the throat with one or both hands. This is the universal sign for choking (see Figure 6-3).

B. If the person cannot answer verbally, or nods the head for yes:

    1. Stand behind the victim.

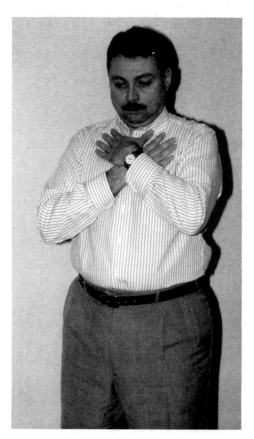

Figure 6-3 The universal sign for choking. Ask "Are you choking?"

2. Reach around the victim's waist, locating the navel. Make a fist and place the thumb side of the fist against the person's abdomen (see Figure 6-4).

3. Grasp your fist with your other hand.

4. Give abdominal thrusts, with the thrusts going in and up at an angle (see Figure 6-5).

C. Repeat the abdominal thrusts until:

1. The object is dislodged and removed.

2. The victim starts to cough or breathe.

3. The victim becomes unconscious.

4. Another medical professional with a higher degree of training takes over.

Unconscious Choking—Adult/Child If the choking victim is unconscious, the individual should be positioned on the back.

A. Check for unresponsiveness.

B. Use the chin lift/head tilt method to open the airway.

C. Give two breaths.

D. If the breaths do not go in, retilt the person's head and give two more breaths. If air still does not go in:

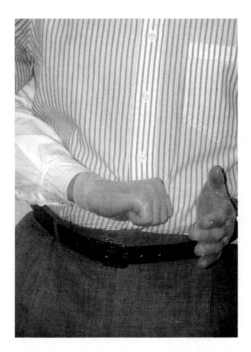

Figure 6-4 Stand behind your victim and find your hand placement.

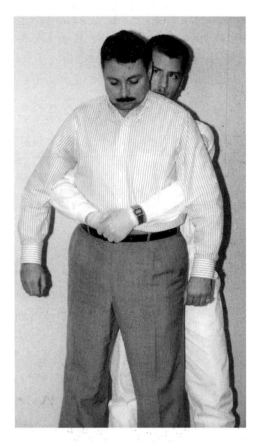

Figure 6-5 Use abdominal thrusts.

1. Straddling the victim's hips is recommended. If you are unable to straddle the victim, kneel next to victim's hips facing them. Be careful not to cause additional injury to the victim.
2. Place heel of one hand just above the navel area.
3. Place the second hand on top of the first hand, keeping the fingers pointed up and off of the rib cage.
4. Give up to 5 abdominal thrusts, keeping the fingers pointed toward the victim's head.

E. Sweep the victim's mouth.

1. Grasp the tongue and lower jaw and lift the jaw.
2. Using the index finger, sweep from one side of the mouth to the other, using a "hook" motion. (If the victim is a child, only sweep if you can see the object.)

3. Give two breaths. If breaths go in:
4. Check for pulse and breathing.
   a. If there is a pulse and no breathing, give rescue breathing.
   b. If there is no pulse and no breathing, administer CPR.
5. If breaths do not go in, repeat abdominal thrusts, finger sweep, and breaths.
6. Follow this procedure until:
   a. The obstruction is cleared.
   b. The person starts to breathe or cough.
   c. Another medical professional with a higher degree of training arrives to take over.

Conscious Infant Infant unable to cry—cyanotic around lips/mouth.

A. Lower infant until head is lower than body.
B. Use 5 sharp back blows between shoulder blades—be sure to support the infant's head by using a C clamp; be sure not to cover the infant's nose or mouth.
C. Turn baby over, lay on table—give 5 chest thrusts; use 2 finger pads; place ring finger just below the nipple line.
D. Repeat until airways cleared and infant is breathing or until the infant becomes unconscious, at which time guidelines for unconscious infant should be followed.

Unconscious Infant

A. Check for unresponsiveness. Tap or gently shake infant's shoulder.
B. If infant does not respond—
C. Look, listen, and feel for 5 seconds.
D. Position infant:
   1. Place on back.
   2. Open airway.
   3. Tilt head/chin back—careful not to tilt it too far back.
   4. Recheck breathing, look, listen, and feel.
E. If infant is not breathing:
   1. Keep head tilted back.
   2. Seal lips over nose and mouth.
   3. Give 2 breaths.

F. If breaths are not accepted:
1. Retilt infant's head and give 2 breaths.
2. Repeat breathing.
G. If breaths still are not accepted
1. Give 5 back blows.
2. Infant's head should be lower than feet.
H. Give 5 chest thrusts.
1. Use 2 finger pads.
2. Place ring fingers just below the nipple line.
3. Place the pads of 2 fingers next to ring finger; raise the ring finger.
I. Do foreign body check.
1. Lift jaw by grasping both tongue and lower jaw of the infant.
2. Attempt to sweep object out only if visible—using the little finger.
J. Tilt head and give 2 breaths. If breaths go in:
1. Check pulse and breathing.
2. If pulse, but no breathing, do rescue breathing.
3. If no pulse or breathing, do CPR.
K. If breaths do not go in:
1. Repeat blows, thrusts, foreign body check, and breathing steps until:
    a. Obstacle is gone.
    b. Infant starts to breathe, cry, or cough.
    c. Other office personnel take over.

Oropharyngeal Airway

The oropharyngeal airway is designed to elevate the tongue away from the oropharynx in the unconscious state (see Figure 6-6). This semi-circular device made from either plastic or rubber prevents the blockage of the airway and allows drainage or suction of secretions. Oropharyngeal airways are to be used on unconscious patients who do not exhibit a gag reflex. The protocol for deciding what patient needs airways should be discussed, and standing orders need to be written that clearly define the guidelines to be used in deciding whether or not the medical personnel can insert the airway.

An airway set should consist of various infant, child, and adult sizes. The procedure for inserting this type of airway is:

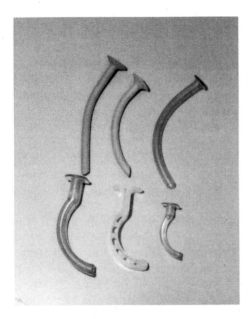

Figure 6-6   Oropharyngeal Airways

1. Select the proper size. There are two ways to measure for correct size. One is to place the airway at the center of the patient's mouth, and it should extend to the angle of the lower jaw. The second way is to hold the device at the corner of the patient's mouth and be sure that it extends to the top of the earlobe on the same side of the face. Never use an airway that is the incorrect size; it can cause vomiting or even force the tongue back to the pharynx.

2. The patient needs to be in the supine position with the head tilted as for ventilation. Use the jaw thrust maneuver if spinal injury is suspected.

3. Open the mouth by crossing the thumb and forefinger, and then scissor open the patient's mouth at the corner.

4. Position airway so that the curved tip is pointing toward the roof of the patient's mouth.

5. Insert the airway. When it touches the soft palate, start to rotate it 180 degrees. Continue until the flange rests on the patient's lips. If it does not touch the lips, remove it.

6. Provide ventilation to the patient.

7. Be alert for the patient's regaining consciousness or attempting to dislodge the airway. Remove the airway by gently pulling it out and down.

Nasopharyngeal Airway

The nasopharyngeal airway is a hollow, curved tube made from soft rubber or plastic. It is to be used on conscious patients who cannot maintain an open airway. Properly positioned, it should extend from the nares down into the oropharynx. It also has a loop at one end that extends around the outside of the nose to prevent slippage into the airway.

The procedure for insertion is:

1. Select the proper size. The airway should approximate the distance from the tip of the patient's nose to the earlobe.

2. Lubricate the airway with a sterile water-soluble gel to decrease irritation to the nasal passage.

3. Using gentle, firm motion, pass the tube into the nostril, sliding the tube into the nose until the lip lies against the flare of the nose. Never force the tube. Remove and try the other nostril.

4. If patient is responsive, have the patient exhale with the mouth closed to assure the tube is in place. Proper insertion will result in air coming through the tube upon exhalation.

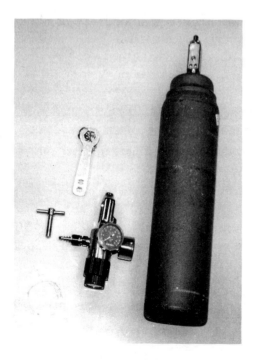

Figure 6-7   Oxygen tank.

Oxygen Therapy

Oxygen is a colorless, odorless gas that is present in the environment at approximately 21 percent.

Pure (100 percent) oxygen can be stored in steel cylinders under pressure of 2,000 pounds per square inch (psi). The cylinders come in various sizes and are labeled with letters. In emergencies, the most commonly used sizes are D, E, and M. The cylinders are also color coded. Oxygen is always stored in green steel cylinders for easy recognition by medical personnel (see Figure 6-7).

The flow of oxygen from the cylinder is controlled by a regulator that reduces the high pressure in the cylinder to a safe range of about 50 psi and controls the flow from 1–15 liters per minute. All regulators have a pressure gauge that measures the pressure within the cylinder. A fresh tank should measure approximately 2,000 psi. Some regulators have a flowmeter that records the flow rate of gas leaving the cylinder. Common safety precautions are listed in Table 6-3.

Administering Oxygen

1. Crack the tank with the wrench supplied, by slowly opening and then closing the cylinder valve to clear it from dust or debris (see Figure 6-8).

2. Check to be sure that the regulator valve is the correct type for the oxygen cylinder and that there is an intact washer.

Table 6-3 Safety Precautions for Oxygen Therapy

1. Protect the cylinder, regulator, fittings, and hoses from combustible materials, like oil or grease.

2. Inspect oxygen level, regulator, fittings, and hoses weekly. A spare tank should be kept in the office.

3. Keep oxygen cylinders secured to the wall in an upright position.

4. Be sure that the regulator valve is the correct size.

5. Keep all valves closed when oxygen cylinder is not in use, even empty cylinders.

6. Always lay the oxygen tank on its side by the patient, with the regulator facing away from the patient's body, to prevent injury to the patient if the regulator valve would blow off.

Remember that there are 2,000 pounds of pressure per square inch in a fresh tank. This is sufficient pressure to remove a patient's head!

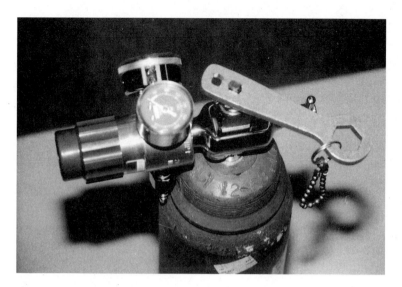

Figure 6-8   Cracking the oxygen tank.

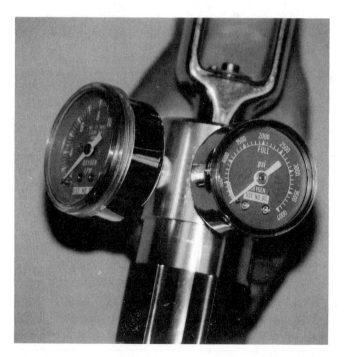

Figure 6-9   Check to make sure there is adequate oxygen in the tank.

3. Apply the regulator valve and tighten securely.

4. Check to be sure that there is an adequate amount of oxygen in the tank—usually at least 200 psi (see Figure 6-9). Open the main cylinder valve slowly about one-half turn beyond the point where the regulator valve becomes pressurized.

5. Check flowmeter to be sure it rises as the valve opens (see Figure 6-10).

6. Attach the tubing or delivery device to the regulator.

7. Attach the delivery device to the patient.

8. Open the control valve to the desired liter flow.

9. When finished administering oxygen to the patient, detach and dispose of delivery system from patient and shut off the control valve until liter flow is at zero.

10. Shut off the main cylinder valve.

11. Open the flowmeter to bleed oxygen out of the system.

12. Detach the regulator by loosening the clamps.

13. Always have the oxygen tank refilled after each use.

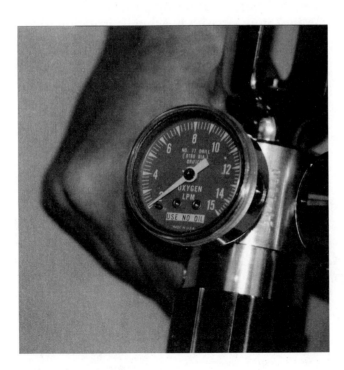

Figure 6-10 Flowmeter.

Devices for Oxygen Delivery

There are a variety of delivery systems to provide oxygen to patients. Each member of the team will need to be familiar with the advantages and disadvantages of each. Supervised training sessions should be conducted to acquaint the office with the proper use of each device. There are 5 basic devices that will be discussed including the nasal cannula, the Venturi mask, the simple face mask, partial and non-rebreathing masks, and the bag valve mask device.

Nasal Cannula

The nasal cannula is used when a low-flow of oxygen is indicated. The room air mixes with the oxygen from the tank. It can deliver 24–40 percent of oxygen at 2–6 liters per minute. The cannula is used for patients with COPD, asthma, emphysema, and uncomplicated heart attack.

The nasal cannula consists of two soft plastic tips inserted a short distance into the nostrils and attached to the cylinder by thin tubing. The nasal cannula and tubing are attached to the oxygen tank, and the liter flow adjusted. Be sure that the oxygen flow can be felt from the nasal prongs. Insert the prongs downward into the patient's nostrils, with the tip facing downward; position the tubing over and behind each ear. Adjust it underneath the chin. If irritation of the cheeks and ears occurs, pad the areas with 2 x 2 gauze (see Figure 6-11).

Venturi Mask

The Venturi mask allows for a more precise measurement of the concentration of inspired oxygen. The mask has adapters that can vary the ultimate concentration of inspired oxygen by altering either the oxygen or air entry from openings. The percentage of oxygen can be controlled by changing adapters that attach to the base of the mask; sometimes an adjustable opening alters the amount of air that can mix with the oxygen. The adapters are marked with the final percentage of delivered oxygen. It ranges from 24–49 percent at 4–8 liters

Table 6-4 Advantages and Disadvantages of the Nasal Cannula

Advantages	Disadvantages
Low-flow oxygen administration.	Drying of mucosa and nares.
Less restrictive than the mask delivery system.	Increased chance for nosebleeds.

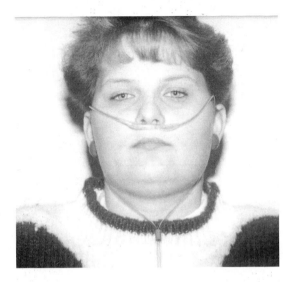

Figure 6-11 Nasal cannula.

per minute. This is the normal range for most systems. This type of system is best used for patients who have chronic obstructive pulmonary disease (COPD).

Simple Face Mask

The simple face mask with an oxygen inlet valve is used to deliver an oxygen concentration ranging from 50–55 percent at liter flow rates of 8–12 liters per minute. It allows a mixture of room air with the oxygen by ports on both sides of the mask, and is used to deliver a moderate concentration of oxygen.

Partial and Non-rebreathing Masks

A partial rebreather mask is one that has a bag attached to it, providing the patient with enriched oxygen during inhalations. The first third of the patient's exhaled air enters the bag, while the remainder leaves through the ports in the sides

Table 6-5 Advantages and Disadvantages of the Venturi Mask

Advantages	Disadvantages
Very precise measurement of delivered oxygen.	Mask is hot and confining, and may irritate the skin.
	Kinking of the tubing may lower oxygen delivery.

Table 6-6   Advantages and Disadvantages of the Simple Face Mask

Advantages	Disadvantages
Eliminates direct contact with the patient's nose and mouth.	Patient complains of feelings of suffocation and tolerates mask poorly.
Can be used to provide rescue breathing to patient.	

of the mask. The non-rebreather works in the same manner except that a one-way valve prevents the exhaled air from entering the reservoir bag. With a tight-fitting mask, this device can result in up to 90 percent oxygen at flow rates of 10–12 liters per minute. It is used primarily for patients who are severely hypoxic but well ventilated. Some conditions are respiratory failure, shock states, and any other condition that causes poor tissue oxygenation. To use the masks and reservoir, first attach the oxygen tubing and provide a flow rate of around 8 liters per minute while keeping a finger over the valve. This action causes the bag to inflate fully. Then apply the mask to the patient's face and secure. Be sure that when the patient inhales the bag does not collapse. If this occurs, increase the deliverance of oxygen by 2-liter increments until the bag remains inflated.

Bag Valve Mask Device

Bag valve masks are self-inflating and can be used without supplemental oxygen. Some masks will have an oxygen attachment port and can deliver 40–69 percent at flow rates of 12 liters per minute. In addition, if a reservoir bag is attached, the concentrates can be increased to almost 100 percent. The mask should fit securely over the patient's chin, beneath the lip, and over the bridge of the nose. It should be transparent and have an air-cushioned rim for sealing.

The bag valve mask can be used for patients who require ventilation (see Figure 6-12). To use this device:

Table 6-7   Advantages and Disadvantages of Partial and Non-rebreathing Mask

Advantages	Disadvantages
Delivers high concentration of oxygen.	Patient complains of feelings of suffocation.

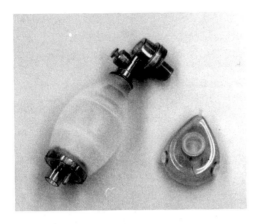

Figure 6-12   Bag valve mask device.

1. Place the patient's head in the chin tilt position.
2. Place mask securely over patient's face. Create a good mask seal by placing the thumb above and the index finger below the valve connection. Hold the patient's jaw with the other finger.

Pediatric Patients

With modifications in size, the devices mentioned above can be used in delivering oxygen to children. Be sure to select the correct size mask and use the appropriate technique when tilting the head. Remember the danger of overinflating the lungs in children. Gastric distention and pneumothorax are

Table 6-8   Advantages and Disadvantages of Bag Valve Mask Device

Advantages	Disadvantages
When used in apneic patients, it allows better control of ventilation and better assessment of how the lungs are responding.	Does not generate the total volume that is possible with mouth-to-mouth ventilation.
Respiratory resistance can be felt as the bag becomes harder to squeeze. Do not continue squeezing bag.	Gastric distention can occur.

possible complications if too much volume is delivered. Monitor the chest movement closely during respiration. Suggested rates of respiration are:

- 0–1 month (newborn):   40–50 breaths/minute.
- 1 month to 1 year (infant):   20–25 breaths/minute.
- 1–8 years (child):   20–25 breaths/minute.

Remember that the above ages are not exact. Gauge the size of the child at the ages listed and act accordingly. If the child remains cyanotic, increase the number of respirations.

Pathophysiology, Signs and Symptoms, Causes, and Emergency Treatment

The ability of the body to deliver sufficient amounts of oxygen to the cells is critical to life. There are many conditions that can interfere with this body function. Medical personnel will deal on a daily basis with patients who suffer from oxygen insufficiency and the resulting complications. Breathing is a function that individuals do without conscious thought until it is brought to their attention. Respiratory conditions make patients very aware of how easily the act of breathing can be compromised. These patients, in particular, are very frightened and require not only medical care but emotional support as well. Remembering to deal with the whole patient, not just the condition, will help to develop trust and understanding between patients and office staff. Some common respiratory conditions seen in the medical office are hyperventilation, COPD (including emphysema, chronic bronchitis, asthma), pneumonia, and acute pulmonary edema.

Hyperventilation

Hyperventilation occurs when an individual breathes rapidly and deeply. The cause can be intentional, as when a swimmer breathes rapidly and deeply before swimming under water, or unintentional, as in psychological stress. It is also seen in cases of aspirin overdose. Most individuals' respiratory rates are determined by the amount of carbon dioxide ions in the bloodstream. An increase in the amount of air entering the lungs results in reduction of carbon dioxide, which eventually leads to a metabolic imbalance called alkalosis. When an individual breathes rapidly and deeply, the carbon dioxide level is lowered. In addition, the pH is altered, causing respiratory alkalosis. Since a normal level of carbon dioxide is needed to maintain the tone of smooth muscle, a drop in carbon dioxide level results in the dilation of blood vessels and a decrease in blood pressure. This condition causes a decrease in the amount of oxygen available to the brain cells and can result in syncope. Patients who are suffering from hyperventilation cannot control their breathing rates. The rapid breathing, in turn, decreases the carbon dioxide level that results in the signs and symptoms associated with this condition.

Signs and Symptoms of Hyperventilation   Signs and symptoms of hyperventilation include:

- Faintness or impaired consciousness and lightheadedness.
- Tightness of the chest and throat.
- Anxiety.
- Blurring of vision.
- Dryness of the mouth.
- A feeling of great tiredness or weakness.
- Palpitation or pounding of the heart.
- Tetany with muscular spasm of the hands and feet (only seen in prolonged attacks).
- Syncope.
- Deep, sighing rapid respiration with rapid pulse.

Before beginning treatment, the office personnel should rule out any organic cause such as diabetic coma, trauma, asthma, or pulmonary embolism.

Treatment of Hyperventilation   The following guidelines should be used to assist the patient in controlling the hyperventilation syndrome.

1. Notify the physician if present.
2. Stay calm and remain non-judgmental. Talk quietly and calmly to the patient.
3. The patient must slow the respiratory rate consciously. Ask the patient to concentrate on breathing slowly.
4. If anxiety has been determined to be the cause of the syndrome, have the patient breathe into an oxygen mask that is not connected to oxygen. Another method that has been used is to have the patient place a finger over one nostril, closing it shut. Another simple method is to have the patient breathe into a brown paper bag.

Chronic Obstructive Pulmonary Disease (COPD)

COPD is a diagnosis given to any pathologic process that decreases the ability of the lung and bronchi to function. In addition, there is permanent damage to the structures of the lungs and bronchi. Diseases most commonly associated with COPD are asthma, chronic bronchitis, and pulmonary emphysema. Many patients seek medical care for these conditions, and medical personnel need to be aware of the causes, signs, symptoms, and treatments of each condition in this category. COPD is the second most common cause of hospitalization in the United States.

Factors contributing to the development of COPD and affecting the degree of severity are cigarette smoking, industrial pollution, allergy, autoimmune genetic predisposition, chronic infections, and exposure to irritating inhalants such as second-hand smoke.

Guidelines for COPD Patients   General guidelines for patients who suffer from COPD should be explained to these patients before an emergency situation occurs. Often the patient is unaware of how much control they could have over the disease process and their ability to function in everyday life. It is the medical personnel's responsibility to educate the patient in the management of the disease. In this chapter, general guidelines are given for the COPD patient, and the diseases categorized under COPD are examined.

1. Explain to the patients why they should stop smoking, avoid other irritating inhalants, take medication as prescribed, and perform ventilation improvement techniques. (Patients who understand are more likely to comply with the medical regimen.)

2. Patients need to be encouraged to follow the exercise program that has been prescribed.

3. Patients with COPD should avoid contact with individuals who have upper respiratory infections. Good personal hygiene and adequate nutrition should be maintained.

4. If ventilation techniques are prescribed, be sure the patient understands the instructions.

5. Patient should be instructed to report any changes in color and amount of sputum.

6. Provide support to the patient and his/her family.

7. Medical personnel should be aware that oxygen therapy should be administered with caution to this patient. Because these patients' stimulus for breathing is based on low oxygen tension, oxygen therapy could remove the stimulus to breathe and result in death. The usual oxygen or-

der is for 24 percent oxygen by Venturi or nasal cannula. **Never administer oxygen without an order from the physician.**

Emphysema

The definition of emphysema is inflation. The terminal bronchioles are plugged with mucus, and air high in carbon dioxide is trapped in the lungs. Permanent enlargement of the air spaces beyond the terminal bronchioles results, as the alveolar walls are destroyed by inadequate oxygen and excessive carbon dioxide. Elasticity of the lungs is lost, which causes more air to be trapped, making breathing difficult especially during the expiratory phase. Cardiomegaly occurs as the heart pumps faster in an attempt to increase the available oxygen to the body systems.

Signs and Symptoms Early signs and symptoms associated with these pathophysiological changes are:

1. Chronic cough (smoker's cough).
2. Shortness of breath.
3. Abnormally rapid breathing.
4. Fatigue.
5. Pursing of the lips during exhalation.

The onset of the disease is chronic, degenerative, and progressive. Patients will experience progressive dyspnea on exertion, chronic cough, and characteristic "barrel chest."

Treatment Patients experiencing severe dyspnea should be examined by the physician. Primary treatment is to relieve the hypoxemia. (See emergency care for chronic bronchitis.)

Chronic Bronchitis

Chronic bronchitis is the inflammation of the bronchial mucous membranes and excessive mucus production in the bronchial tree. Bronchitis can be acute or chronic. Chronic bronchitis is indicated by repeated attacks of acute bronchitis and coughing, with sputum production that lasts several months over at least 2 consecutive years.

The continuous obstruction of respiratory passages and increased secretion from the bronchial mucosa reduce the amount of air entering the alveoli. Repeated infections result in scar tissue that further narrows the bronchi.

Signs and Symptoms Signs and symptoms of chronic bronchitis are:

1. Chronic cough with sputum production.
2. Weight gain due to edema.
3. Cyanosis.
4. Tachypnea.
5. Wheezing.
6. Chest pain.
7. Fever.

Treatment The emergency treatment of both emphysema and chronic bronchitis is providing oxygen to the patient. The major threat to life in COPD is a lack of oxygen. However, these patients breathe because oxygen levels have become too low. Too much oxygen will result in apnea. The order to administer oxygen should be given by the physician. In the absence of the physician, standing orders can be written for medical personnel to follow.

Treatment of these patients calls for assisting the breathing process:

1. Establish an airway.
2. Position patient in an upright or semi-Fowler's position to facilitate breathing.
3. Administer oxygen slowly through nasal cannula at 2–4 liters per minute.
4. Monitor patient's respiratory rate and depth. Watch patient closely.
5. Continue to increase the oxygen flow every 5 minutes until cyanosis clears.
6. Maintain body temperature.
7. Loosen any restrictive clothing.
8. Reassure the patient and family members.

Asthma

Asthma is the Greek word for panting. Within the respiratory system, there is a blockage of the bronchi due to a sudden contraction of the smooth muscle in the walls of the bronchi. This spasm narrows the lumen of the tubes, making breathing, particularly expiration, difficult. In addition, the mucous membrane becomes swollen with fluid, further narrowing the lumen. Stale air becomes trapped, reducing the amount of air that can enter the lungs. A characteristic wheezing sound is produced.

The causes of the spasms are varied. Often there is a family history of allergy and the patient will have a history of hypersensitivity. Upper respiratory infection, exercise, and psychological stress can bring on an attack.

Asthma causes approximately 6,000 deaths every year in the United States. Asthma occurs before age 10 in about half of all cases; 95 percent of all chronic asthma is seen in children. The patient experiences acute attacks with periods of being asymptomatic.

Asthma can be divided into three classifications according to cause (see Table 6-9). Extrinsic asthma is caused by an allergy to antigens such as pollen, dust, and smoke. Intrinsic asthma is usually secondary to chronic bronchitis, sinusitis, tonsillitis, or adenoiditis. The third classification is mixed, which is a combination of extrinsic and intrinsic factors.

Signs and Symptoms Signs and symptoms of asthma include:

1. Dyspnea.
2. Patient assumes upright position.
3. Profuse perspiration.
4. Tachypnea.
5. Tightness in the chest.
6. Rapid pulse.

Table 6-9 Three Classifications of Asthma

Type	Cause	Population	Seasonal
Extrinsic	Allergies to pollen and dust.	One half are children.	Spring/fall.
Intrinsic	Viral infections, cold air, emotion, inhaled fumes. Believed to be caused by hypersensitivity to the bacteria causing the infection.	Adults.	None.
Mixed	Usually has childhood asthma that the patient does not "grow out of."	Children/adults.	

7. Rapid, shallow respirations.
8. Fatigue.

Treatment of Acute Attack To treat an acute attack:

1. Notify the physician.
2. Establish an open airway.
3. Administer high-flow, humidified oxygen. The moisture will help to loosen secretions.
4. Help the patient to remain calm. Remember that stress and emotions worsen an attack.
5. If patient has no condition that contraindicates it, such as renal failure or congestive heart failure, force fluids.
6. Epinephrine and aminophylline may be ordered by the physician.

Status Asthmaticus Asthma attacks can occur that are severe and prolonged. This condition is called SA, a life-threatening emergency requiring immediate attention. Signs and symptoms may include:

1. Overinflated chest.
2. Tachycardia.
3. Exhaustion.
4. Dehydration.
5. Extremely labored breathing.

Treatment of Status Asthmatics Follow the guidelines for the acute asthma attack and, in addition:

1. Call EMS.
2. Monitor vital signs.
3. Follow established office protocol.

Pneumonia

There are at least 50 different types of pneumonia. It is the fifth leading cause of death in the United States. The cause of pneumonia is inflammation of the lungs resulting in congestion and condensation. Structures affected are the bronchioles, alveolar ducts, alveolar sacs, and alveoli of the lungs. The inflammation can occur unilaterally or bilaterally. Classification of pneumonia is based upon cause—bacterial (diplococci pneumonia), viral, chemical, bronchial, or lobar pneumonia. Another cause can be the inhalation of foreign objects into the lungs, which is called aspiration pneumonia.

Signs and Symptoms Signs and symptoms are chest pain, dyspnea, rapid respiration, respiratory distress, productive cough, rhonchi, fever, chills, hot and dry skin, orthopnea.

Emergency Treatment
1. Notify the physician.
2. Position the patient in an upright or semi-Fowler's position.
3. If ordered, administer oxygen at 50–100 percent by mask.
4. Loosen restrictive clothing.
5. Stay with patient.

Pulmonary Edema

Pulmonary edema is the accumulation of fluid in lung tissue and within the alveoli. This is commonly caused by the inhalation of irritating gases, congestive heart failure, diffuse infections, barbiturate and opiate poisoning, and renal failure.

Causes other than cardiogenic are aspiration pneumonia, smoke inhalation, or near-drowning patients.

Signs and Symptoms Signs and symptoms of pulmonary edema are:

1. Dyspnea.
2. Crackling or wheezing sounds.
3. Cyanosis.
4. Rapid pulse.
5. Anxiety.
6. Distended jugular vein (patient is struggling to draw in oxygen).
7. Restlessness (due to lack of oxygen)
8. Orthopnea—patient can breathe only in an upright position, not lying down.

Emergency Treatment Emergency treatment for pulmonary edema is:

1. Notify physician immediately and/or call EMS.
2. Establish airway.
3. On physician's order, administer high-flow oxygen.

4. Elevate patient's head and shoulders.
5. Keep patient still and calm.

Summary

Health care professionals need to be able to deal with life-threatening respiratory emergencies immediately. A general understanding of how the respiratory system functions, what devices are necessary, and how to deliver oxygen are necessary skills. Training should be obtained on how to perform rescue breathing and on how to deal with a choking patient.

The diseases associated with this system can be acute or chronic, progressive, and debilitating for patients. In addition, when the ability to breathe is impaired, health care professionals must be prepared to deal with the psychological aspects of the situation.

Review Questions

1. Which type of airway is used for the following patient?
   The patient is a 38-year-old male; blood pressure is 120/80, respiration 40, wheezing, cyanotic, pupils dilated, and the victim is conscious.
2. Explain why it is necessary to take a CPR course from a trained instructor.
3. List the 6 safety precautions for the use of oxygen.
4. Give the criteria for using the following devices:
   - Nasal cannula.
   - Venturi mask.
   - Simple face mask.
   - Partial and non-rebreathing mask.
   - Bag valve mask device.
5. Explain why hyperventilation occurs.
6. How can you assist the patient in controlling hyperventilation?
7. What does COPD mean?
8. List the diseases most commonly associated with COPD, and identify the signs and symptoms of each.
9. Explain the 7 guidelines for dealing with the COPD patient.

10. List the signs and symptoms associated with emphysema.
11. What pathophysiological changes occur with chronic bronchitis?
12. Explain the emergency treatment for:
    - Chronic bronchitis.
    - Asthma.
    - Pneumonia.
13. How and why does asthma occur?
14. Define status asthmaticus.

CHAPTER 7

Cardiovascular Diseases

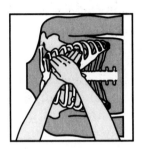

Objectives

After completing this chapter the learner should be able to:

1. Describe the function of the cardiovascular system.

2. Describe how to assess the patient for cardiac distress.

3. Describe the cause of coronary artery disease.

4. List the cause, signs, symptoms, and treatment of myocardial infarction.

5. List the cause, signs, symptoms, and treatment of congestive heart failure.

6. Identify and describe the steps and appropriate procedure necessary to perform CPR.

7. Describe the steps that should take place following an emergency.

Introduction

Cardiovascular disease is the number one killer in the United States today. Approximately 30 million Americans have some form of heart disease. Of these, one-half million will die this year before they reach the hospital. Patients who complain of chest pain should always be treated as heart attack victims until diagnosed otherwise.

Diseases of the heart can affect the layers of the heart and the endocardium within the heart. These structures may be affected separately or together. While the types and causes of heart disease are many, the effects are few. Because the heart's primary action is to pump blood, a diseased heart often fails to pump blood efficiently. This failure in turn affects each system as the blood available to the body is compromised. Often these diseases start within the arteries and progress if left untreated.

The most common cause of severe heart problems begins as coronary artery disease, which can lead to angina pectoris and may lead to acute myocardial infarction. Certain risk factors have been identified that predispose individuals to these disease processes. There are risk factors that can be controlled, such as smoking, high cholesterol, stress, hypertension, diabetes, and a lack of exercise. Patients should be encouraged to take charge of these factors and reduce the risk of heart disease. There are also risk factors that patients have no control over, such as hereditary traits, gender (males are more likely to be affected than females), age, and race (African Americans are more prone to hypertension).

Anatomical Overview

The major function of the heart is to pump blood. It is a muscular organ about the size of a fist, located in the center of the chest with 2/3 of it lying on the left side. Blood moves through the heart in one direction. The right side of the heart receives the unoxygenated blood and delivers it to the lungs. The left side of the heart receives the oxygenated blood from the lungs and pumps it out to the body. The four-chambered muscular organ receives unoxygenated blood from the superior and inferior vena cava, then circulates it to the lungs where it picks up oxygen and drops off carbon dioxide to be exhaled. Oxygenated blood returns to the heart and is "pumped" out through the major artery called the aorta. It continues flowing to the arteries and eventually reaches all body cells (see Figures 7-1 and 7-2).

The pumping action is regulated by an electrical conduction system within the heart tissue. The sinoatrial (SA) node, sometimes called the pacemaker, fires an electrical impulse, which spreads to the atrioventricular (AV) node and also causes the top two chambers of the heart (the atria) to contract. The impulse continues across to the bundle of His located between the two lower chambers (the ventricles). The impulse continues down the bundle branches on either side of the septum and then goes out to the network called the Purkinje fibers, resulting in the contraction of the ventricles (see Figure 7-3).

The heart receives blood through its own arteries. Three main coronary arteries are the first to branch off the aorta and provide nourishment to the heart.

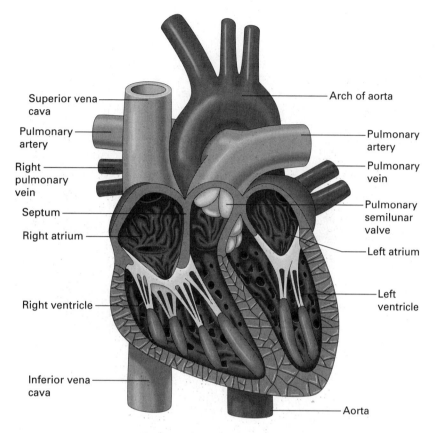

Heart—Pulmonary Arteries and Veins

Figure 7-1   Heart—pulmonary arteries and veins.

They are the right coronary artery, the left coronary artery, and the anterior descending branch (which comes off the left coronary artery).

Pathophysiology, Signs and Symptoms, Causes, and Emergency Treatment

Coronary Artery Disease

Coronary artery disease occurs when the vessels of the heart become occluded. The occlusion can be caused by a blood clot forming in the inner walls of the coronary artery, causing a coronary thrombosis, or from a narrowing of the lumen within the vessel. Atherosclerosis is the condition in which the narrowing

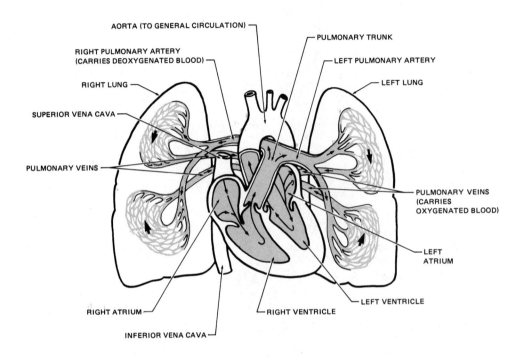

AORTA (TO GENERAL CIRCULATION)

PULMONARY TRUNK

RIGHT PULMONARY ARTERY
(CARRIES DEOXYGENATED BLOOD)

LEFT PULMONARY ARTERY

RIGHT LUNG

LEFT LUNG

SUPERIOR VENA CAVA

PULMONARY VEINS

PULMONARY VEINS
(CARRIES
OXYGENATED BLOOD)

LEFT
ATRIUM

LEFT VENTRICLE

RIGHT ATRIUM

RIGHT VENTRICLE

INFERIOR VENA CAVA

Figure 7-2 Pulmonary circulation.

of the lumen is caused by deposits of fatty material in the bends of the arteries (see Figure 7-4). This narrowing restricts the blood flow to the area of the heart supplied by the occluded artery and can continue narrowing until the artery is totally blocked, resulting in a myocardial infarction. Partial blockage of the artery can result in a condition known as angina pectoris.

Angina Pectoris

Angina pectoris is a clinical syndrome that often accompanies arteriosclerotic heart disease. It is chest pain caused by the narrowing of the arteries, resulting in arteriospasm. The heart must have a constant supply of oxygenated blood in order to function. This narrowing of arteries allows only a limited amount of oxygen to be delivered to the heart. Angina attacks can be caused by any condition that increases myocardial oxygen demand, such as stress, eating, exertion, or even, in susceptible individuals, extremes of temperature and humidity.

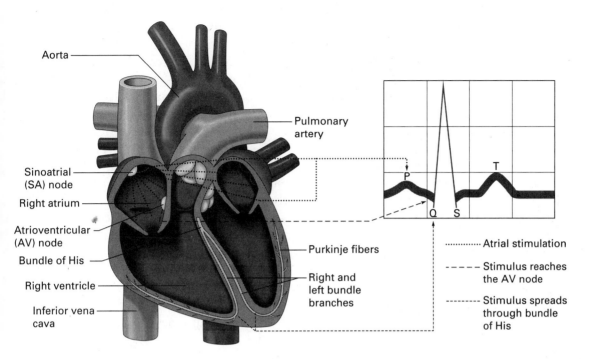

Figure 7-3 Conduction system of the heart showing the source of electrical impulses.

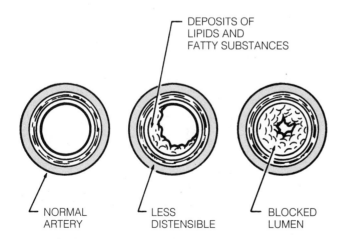

Figure 7-4 Atherosclerosis of the artery.

Signs and Symptoms Angina pectoris may be described as severe substernal chest pain or a feeling of tightness, squeezing, burning, and pressure. Nausea, vomiting, and shortness of breath may also be present. The pain is located on the left side of the chest in about 90 percent of the patients. Sometimes the pain will radiate up to the upper and lower jaws and down the arms and shoulder blade. Attacks usually last less than 15 minutes and no more than 30 minutes.

Because the blood supply to the heart is compromised by narrow arteries, increased demands for oxygen by the heart often cannot be met. As the heart pumps faster in response to a factor, not enough oxygen can be delivered to meet the increased demand by the cardiac cells, resulting in pain (angina pectoris). This pain can be relieved by rest, shortly after the patient stops all activity. The patient may have already been prescribed a vasodilator called nitroglycerin. These tablets or patches dilate the coronary arteries to increase the blood flow to the heart, eliminating or reducing the pain. Tablets are used sublingually (placed under the tongue) for rapid results.

These attacks are reversible and leave no damage to the heart. However, the attacks are an indication of cardiac problems, and patients should be instructed to inform the office of all attacks that occur. In addition, patient and family education should be provided. Angina attacks and myocardial infarctions are impossible for the layperson to tell apart.

Major Risk Factors The majority of patients who have angina are men in their 50s and 60s. Major risk factors for the development of angina are:

- Presence of coronary artery disease.
- Smoking (cigarettes, cigars, pipes).
- Obesity.
- Stress.
- Hypertension.

All patients who call the office complaining of chest pain need to be seen immediately by medical personnel.

Emergency Treatment Patients with chest pain require the following care:

1. Notify the physician.
2. Patient is to cease all movement.
3. Place patient in semi-reclining or sitting position.
4. If patient has prescribed nitroglycerin, instruct patient to place 1 tablet underneath the tongue. Tablets may be taken every 5 minutes up to 15

minutes. If pain persists, the possibility of heart attack is likely. (If physician is present, follow office protocol.)

5. With physician's order, administer high-flow oxygen via mask to patient.
6. Loosen restrictive clothing.
7. Maintain body temperature.
8. **Never leave the patient alone.** Talk to the patient to give reassurance.
9. Monitor vital signs. Administer CPR if cardiac arrest occurs.
10. If physician is not present in the office, call EMS.

Myocardial Infarction

Myocardial infarctions, often called heart attacks, occur when the blood flow is severely reduced or completely stopped to the heart. This loss of oxygen to the heart results in necrosis of heart tissue. This ischemia can result from any of the following:

1. Congestive heart failure, which usually develops 3–7 days after a previous MI. Blood backs up into the lungs because the heart is not pumping efficiently.
2. Cardiac arrhythmia. Because of injury to the heart and/or the electrical conduction system of the heart, the heart beats in an irregular fashion.

Sudden Death   A half million people in the United States die within two hours of the onset of a myocardial infarction. This occurrence requires administering prompt and swift medical care to these people.

Myocardial infarction can be caused by a thrombosis or clot occluding the coronary artery, or from a spasm in the coronary arteries. Less frequently, the heart is not able to meet its own demands for oxygen over an extended period of time.

Whatever the cause, the signs and symptoms of myocardial infarction must be responded to immediately. This is a life-threatening situation. When office personnel are in doubt about the cause of the patient's symptoms, it is safe to proceed as if the patient is experiencing an MI.

Signs and Symptoms   Common signs and symptoms are:

■ Chest pain can be described as crushing, tightness in the chest, or squeezing of the chest. Patients will not always describe this as pain, but rather a discomfort or a feeling of pressure.

- Pain can occur in the arms, neck, jaw area, and/or scapular area on either side of the body.
- Nausea.
- Vomiting.
- Shortness of breath.
- Diaphoresis.
- Cyanosis.
- Anxiety.
- Patient denial of the possibility of a heart attack occurring.
- Bradycardia—pulse less than 60.
- Hypotension.

Medical personnel should remember that patients who suffer from angina pectoris will have similar symptoms. As a general rule, however, angina attacks will subside after the patient ceases all activities, and the pain is usually of a short duration. Typically, the pain caused by a myocardial infarction lasts longer than 2 minutes and, while it may come and go, never truly stops. Angina patients need to be encouraged to keep track of their attacks because they usually increase in number shortly before a myocardial infarction. All patients who call the office complaining of chest pain need medical attention.

Never put these patients on hold! Immediately notify the physician and proceed with office protocol.

Emergency Treatment This treatment is intended as a general guideline for the care of a myocardial infarction patient. Medical office staff should discuss and document their own office protocol for dealing with this emergency.

1. Notify the physician and/or EMS.
2. Assess for ABCs (airway, breathing, and circulation).
3. Keep patient immobile and remain at patient's side. Place patient in semi-Fowler's position.
4. Crash drawer should be brought to the patient's side.
5. Loosen restrictive clothing.
6. Maintain body temperature.
7. Monitor vital signs every 5 minutes or more often if indicated.
8. One office staff member should document care given and vital signs as taken.

9. If ordered, administer oxygen at 6 liters per minute by face mask.
10. Offer support to the patient and family members.

These patients and their families are often very anxious. Be sure that psychological first aid is given as well as physical. The patient may want to know if this is a heart attack. Be sure that any diagnosis made comes from the physician, not the office staff. By remaining calm and explaining why the care is being given, the compliance of the patient and family members can be increased.

Congestive Heart Failure (CHF)

CHF occurs when the heart fails to pump enough blood to meet the body's needs. Circulatory congestion results, either as systemic venous circulation resulting in peripheral edema, or pulmonary circulation congestion resulting in pulmonary edema—an acute life-threatening condition. This heart failure is a result of many cardiac and pulmonary disease processes. Acute congestive heart failure usually results from a myocardial infarction.

Signs and Symptoms Signs and symptoms of CHF will differ according to the side of the heart where the congestion occurs. Left-sided or pulmonary circulation congestion results in shortness of breath (dyspnea). Right-sided or systemic venous circulation results in distended neck veins, hepatomegaly, and edema.

Because CHF is a progressive condition, advanced CHF may include tachypnea, heart palpitation, edema, diaphoresis, cyanosis, anxiety, mild to severe confusion, and increased blood pressure.

Emergency Treatment
1. Notify the physician and/or activate EMS.
2. Have the patient sit up with feet dangling. This position helps the fluid to settle in the extremities and not the lungs.
3. If ordered, administer 100 percent high-flow oxygen by mask.
4. Follow office protocol.

Cardiopulmonary Resuscitation (CPR)

Cardiopulmonary resuscitation is a method providing artificial circulation. It increases the survival rate of a victim of cardiac arrest by combining chest compression and rescue breathing to provide the oxygen necessary for the continuing function of body cells. Without delivered oxygen, brain cells will start to die within 4–6 minutes. This is called biological death and is irreversible.

The CPR method will only deliver about 1/3 of the normal blood to the brain; therefore, it alone is not enough to help the cardiac arrest patient survive. EMS should be notified immediately and CPR begun immediately if indicated. Any delay will reduce the survival rate. Be aware, as health professionals, that CPR does not guarantee a patient will survive. If the heart is too damaged, no amount of CPR will help the patient. Be prepared for failure and the resulting death of the patient. Knowing what to do and executing the sequential steps in CPR should assure the professional that everything was done that could be done.

Before attempting CPR, medical personnel should have taken a course from a certified instructor in order to learn the correct technique. It is not good enough to just know the steps; one should be able to perform correctly the techniques involved.

CPR Procedure

A. Establish unresponsiveness. Tap or gently shake the patient (see Figure 7-5). Be sure to do both actions as some patients may be hard of hearing or deaf.

B. Look, listen, feel. Lean over patient with rescuer's face toward patient's feet.

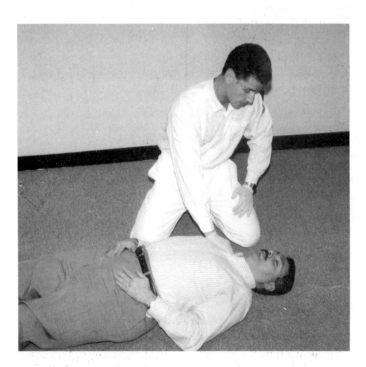

Figure 7-5   Checking for unresponsiveness.

1. Look to see if chest is moving.
2. Listen for air leaving the lungs.
3. Feel for breath.

C. If not breathing, position properly. Position patient on firm, flat surface with head even with the heart. Patient should be in supine position.

    1. If patient is on the abdomen or side, log roll the patient onto the back. Be careful to move body as a unit if there are suspected spinal injuries.

    2. CPR should not be attempted on any surface other than firm and flat.

D. Airway.

    1. Tilt head back by placing the hand on the patient's head and pushing back.

    2. Lift chin by placing two fingers on the bony part of the chin and lifting (see Figure 7-6).

    3. This technique opens the airway; breathing should be rechecked. The tongue is the number one cause of airway obstruction, and this method causes the tongue to fall back out of the way.

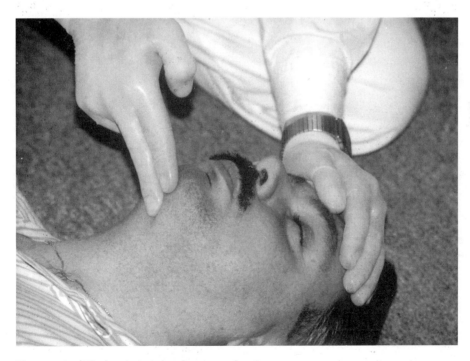

Figure 7-6   Tilt the victim's head to open the airway.

4. If a spinal injury is suspected, use the modified jaw thrust method.

E. Look, listen, feel (see Figure 7-7), for 5 seconds.

F. If breathing is absent:

1. Keep head tilted back; pinch nose closed.

2. Seal patient's mouth with a mouthpiece.

3. Give 2 slow breaths.

a. Each should last 1 1/2 seconds.

b. Patient's chest should rise.

c. Lift off mouth in between breaths.

G. Pulse

1. Check for pulse at the carotid artery.

2. Find Adam's apple; slide fingers down in groove of neck closest to you (see Figure 7-8).

3. Check pulse for 5–10 seconds. If no pulse—

H. Position hands on chest.

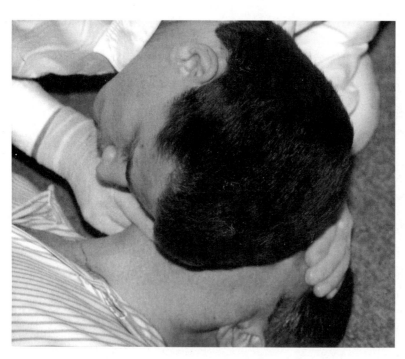

Figure 7-7 Look, listen, and feel for breathing.

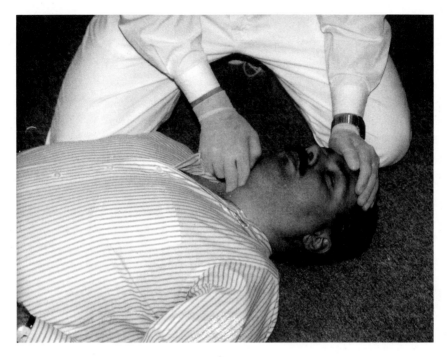

Figure 7-8   Check for the carotid pulse.

1. Locate the xiphoid process with the hand closest to patient's feet (notch at the lower end of the sternum). Place two fingers above the notch (see Figures 7-9 and 7-10).
2. Place heel of the hand closest to patient's head on the sternum next to, but not touching, the fingers.
3. Lift hand closest to patient's feet and place on top of other hand (see Figure 7-11).
4. Be sure to keep the fingers off the chest area.
5. Straighten the elbows. Position shoulders directly over hands (see Figure 7-12).

I. Compressions:
   1. Compress the sternum 1 1/2 to 2 in. Be sure to use a smooth, even downward push. Don't rock.
   2. Count out loud to 15 compressions. This should take around 10 seconds.
   3. Be sure hands remain on the chest the entire time when delivering compressions and between compressions.

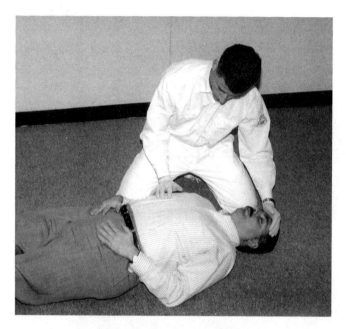

Figure 7-9   Run your fingers up the rib cage until you find the notch at the bottom of the sternum.

J. Two slow breaths.
   1. Open airway (head tilt/chin lift).
   2. Seal patient's mouth with a mouthpiece.
   3. Give 2 slow breaths lasting around 1 1/2 seconds.
   4. Be sure chest rises with each breath; rescuer should lift mouth off patient's between breaths.
K. Repeat compression/breathing cycles. Repeat 15 compressions/2 breaths.
L. Recheck the pulse.
   1. After 1 minute of CPR, recheck pulse for 5 seconds.
   2. If pulse is present and patient is breathing:
      a. Stay with patient.
      b. Keep airway open.
      c. Monitor breathing.
   3. If pulse is present but breathing is not, do rescue breathing.
   4. If person does not have a pulse and is not breathing, continue with compression/breathing. Recheck pulse every few minutes.

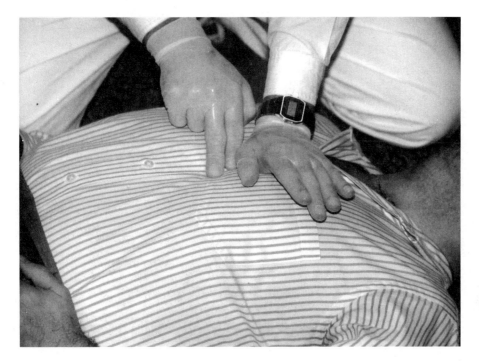

Figure 7-10 Place two fingers above the notch, with the heel of the other hand above the fingers. Take care to stay above the notch.

When to Stop CPR

Once CPR is initiated, there are only four reasons CPR should be stopped.

1. Heart starts beating adequately on its own.
2. Victim and rescuer become endangered at the site.
3. Another trained individual takes over.
4. Rescuer becomes exhausted and can no longer continue.

CPR is intended as an emergency procedure to maintain cellular oxygen perfusion until more advanced care can be given. Always remember that CPR should be started immediately after the cardiac arrest and should not be interrupted unless certain specific conditions exist.

Infant and Child CPR

Infant and child CPR differ slightly from the adult technique. Modification is made in speed and strength of breathing/compression. See Table 7-1 for comparison of infant, child, and adult CPR.

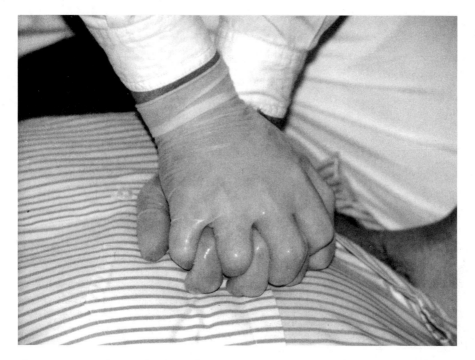

Figure 7-11 Lock your fingers and prepare to give chest compressions. Be sure fingers are not on the ribs.

Following the Emergency

The office personnel will need to assess their response to these emergencies by asking and answering the following questions. Did personnel follow office protocol? Were there any difficulties observed in delivering the care? Were office personnel and equipment adequately prepared and ready to deal with these life-threatening emergencies? An office meeting or session should be held to allow the staff to discuss their fears and concerns about the emergency. Cardiac emergencies are likely to occur frequently in the medical office, due to the large number of patients who have heart diseases. The office personnel who are trained to spot potential cardiac problems and deal effectively with these emergencies can save lives.

Summary

As the general population grows older, and the American diet remains high in fat, medical staff will continue to see more cardiac patients in the office. Cardiovascular disease is the number one cause of death for Americans, and med-

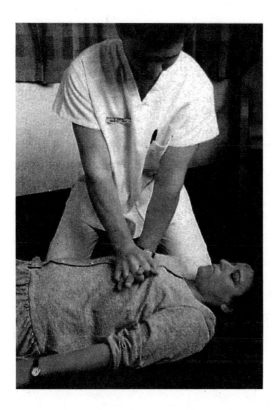

Figure 7-12 Position your body so that spreading of the knees gives a support base, lean with your shoulders directly over the victim, lock elbows, and give chest compressions. (From Krebs and Wise, *Medical Assisting, Clinical Competencies,* © 1994, Delmar Publishers.)

Table 7-1　CPR Comparison Chart

	Adult	Child	Infant
Breathing	2 breaths, then 2 breaths every 15 compressions.	2 breaths initially, then 1 every 5 compressions.	2 breaths initially, then 1 every 5 compressions.
Compression	15 compressions, 1 1/2–2in. depth.	5 compressions, 1–1 1/2in. depth.	5 compressions, 1/2–1in. depth (check pulse at brachial artery).
Rate	15 compressions in around 10 seconds.	5 compressions in around 4 seconds.	5 compressions in around 4 seconds.
Hand Position	One hand on top of the lower 1/2 of sternum.	Use one hand on lower 1/2 of sternum.	Two fingers on lower 1/2 of sternum.
		Keep other hand on forehead.	Position directly below nipple line. Keep other hand on forehead.

ical offices need to be prepared to deal with this type of patient. All office personnel should be trained in CPR and in how to recognize the classic symptoms of cardiac difficulties. Responding quickly and efficiently will save the lives of many patients.

Review Questions

1. If the electrical conduction system of the heart is disrupted, what occurs?

2. A patient sitting in the examination room complains of chest pain, nausea, sweating, and cyanosis. What should the medical office personnel do? How does the situation change if the patient telephones the complaint to the office?

3. Explain why psychological first aid is as important as physical first aid with a cardiac patient.

4. What occurs in left-sided CHF? Right-sided CHF?

5. You have just experienced the death of an MI patient. What should take place in the staff meeting?

CHAPTER 8

Bleeding/Hemorrhage

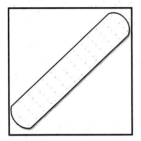

Objectives

After completing this chapter the learner should be able to:

1. Describe the function of blood.
2. Differentiate between arterial and venous bleeding.
3. Locate the appropriate pressure points to control bleeding.
4. List the signs and symptoms of internal bleeding.
5. Differentiate between the different types of wounds.
6. Identify appropriate first aid for the different types of wounds.
7. List the dangers associated with bleeding.

Introduction

The average adult human body contains approximately 6 liters of blood, comprising about 8 percent of body weight. Loss of 1 liter or more of blood can be life threatening. Efforts must be made to minimize blood loss without putting the patient at additional risk. In order to maximize patient care, it is important for medical personnel to understand the function of blood and how it works to maintain optimal body physiology.

Anatomical Overview

Blood acts as the transportation system of the body. It carries oxygen and nutrients to all body cells so that they can perform their individual functions. It transports toxic byproducts of the body to various locations for excretion. Blood cells are a major part of the immune system. These cells work to protect the body from a variety of microorganisms. Blood also helps to maintain body temperature. Blood is comprised of two major elements: plasma and formed elements. Plasma is the fluid that carries these elements throughout the body for dispersion. Red blood cells carry oxygen throughout the body to aid in cellular metabolism, and they carry carbon dioxide to the lungs for excretion from the body. White blood cells function to protect the body from foreign organisms. Platelets are essential for normal blood clotting and help to control blood loss from broken vessels.

The body maintains approximately 60,000 miles of blood vessels in various sizes to accommodate the different body locations and needs. In comparison, this would approximate a little more than 10 round trips by car between San Francisco and New York City. It takes approximately 70 seconds for blood to make one complete circuit throughout the body.

The heart is the central pumping unit for the blood and controls volume dispersement. Oxygen-rich blood is pumped from the heart through the arteries and travels through the capillaries. Oxygen-poor blood is returned to the heart through the venous system.

Bleeding

There are two basic categories of injuries that cause bleeding: external and internal. External bleeding is caused by an injury that breaks the continuity of the skin. Internal bleeding is caused by damage to internal body tissue.

There are three types of bleeding: arterial bleeding, venous bleeding, and capillary oozing.

Arterial Bleeding

When there is a break in the continuity of the structure that is known as the artery, bleeding tends to be rapid and profuse. Bright red blood will spurt from this type of wound with each beat of the heart. This type of bleeding is immediately life-threatening. Blood from a damaged artery will not usually clot because the blood flow is too forceful. The exception would be if the artery is very

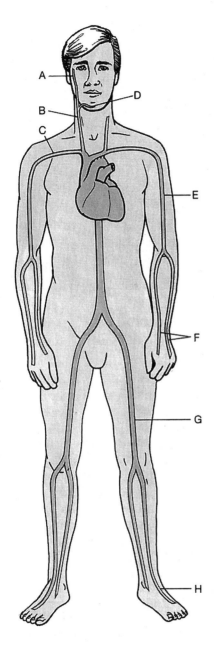

Figure 8-1 Pressure points: (A) temporal artery, (B) carotid artery, (C) subclavian artery, (D) facial artery, (E) brachial artery, (F) radial artery, (G) femoral artery, (H) dorsalis pedis (From Krebs and Wise, *Medical Assisting, Clinical Competencies,* © 1994, Delmar Publishers.)

small, in which case the blood would clot and bleeding would cease. Because arteries have the ability to constrict and dilate, a completely severed artery could seal itself in the event of traumatic amputation.

Venous Bleeding

Bleeding from a damaged vein will be less forceful than arterial bleeding, smoother flowing, and a darker red in color. Because the bleeding is less forceful, clotting will be more likely and bleeding will be easier to control.

Capillary Oozing

When capillaries are damaged, bleeding is much less intense than either arterial or venous bleeding; the blood from capillary oozing is light red in color. Clotting typically occurs within 2–6 minutes. There is little danger of capillary blood loss causing a threat to life, but wound contamination and potential infection is a danger.

Hemophilia

While the average individual's blood does clot within 2–6 minutes, if an individual has hemophilia, or "bleeder's disease," the blood clotting mechanism is faulty and the blood will not clot. Medical personnel should be aggressive in their attempt to stop the bleeding, using appropriate first-aid measures, in addition to activating the EMS system as quickly as possible. An individual with hemophilia can bleed to death from minor wounds.

External Bleeding Control Techniques

In dealing with external bleeding, the methods to be used are:

- Direct pressure on the wound.
- Elevation.
- Pressure on the supplying artery.
- Pressure bandage.
- Tourniquet (to be used only as a last resort technique).

Direct Pressure

Any time medical personnel are dealing with visible blood (or other body fluids), latex gloves should to be worn to protect the caregiver from contracting a possible blood-borne pathogen, and also to protect the patient from exposure to possible contaminants. Direct pressure involves placing a sterile dressing or the cleanest material available against the bleeding area and pressing firmly with the heel of the hand until a bandage can be applied. If blood soaks through the dressing, simply apply additional dressings on top of the blood-soaked dressing and continue to apply pressure. Any attempt to remove dressings already in place may disturb the formation of a blood clot and may increase bleeding. Other medical personnel will need to alert the physician if one is not immediately present. In cases where the physician is absent, the safest measure is to activate the EMS system if the wound is large and bleeding is profuse.

Elevation

In addition to direct pressure on the wound, the injured limb should be elevated above the level of the heart. If there is the suspicion of a fracture, dislocation, or spinal injury, **DO NOT** elevate or move the injured part.

Pressure on the Supplying Artery

Wounds where the bleeding is not controlled by direct pressure and elevation will require more aggressive methods. Pressure on the supplying artery consists of using three fingers to apply pressure on the brachial artery or the heel of the hand to apply pressure to the femoral artery in an effort to control bleeding. Pressure points are in those areas of the body where the artery lies close to a bony structure near the skin surface. The pressure that is supplied causes the artery to be compressed against the underlying bony structure and slows the blood flow to the wound area. This reduced flow gives the blood an opportunity to clot.

Criteria for using this method of blood control include:

- Continuing with direct pressure and elevation.
- There is no suspicion of damage to the underlying bone.
- Never apply this method of control to the carotid artery. This type of pressure could result in cardiac arrhythmia and/or cardiac arrest.

Pressure Points While there are 8 basic pressure points that can be utilized, the brachial and femoral arteries are the most often used and will be explained in detail (see Figure 8-1). Medical personnel should be able to locate and occlude these arteries quickly and effectively.

Brachial Artery The brachial artery is located in the groove on the inside of the arm halfway between the axilla and the elbow. To apply pressure, grasp the upper middle arm from below with the thumb on the outside of the arm. The fingers should be located on the inside of the upper arm. Using the flat inside surface of the fingers, apply pressure to compress the brachial artery against the humerus. Remember that the direct pressure and elevation should not be discontinued. This pressure point is used to control bleeding in the upper extremities.

Femoral Artery This pressure point is located at the front middle part of the crease in the groin area, usually where the elastic of underwear lies. To apply pressure, position the patient on the back. If possible, kneel next to the opposite side of the body from the wound. Place the heel of one hand directly on the pressure point (in the crease of the groin) and lean forward to apply pressure. Additional pressure can be added by using both hands if necessary to control bleeding. Using the heel of one hand, apply pressure directly to the artery, place the heel of the other hand on top of the fingertips, and lean forward.

Pressure Bandages

In cases where the patient has multiple wound areas or needs additional attention, a pressure bandage can be applied. The pressure bandage is used to hold the dressing in place and to help control bleeding. While dressings need to be sterile, bandages need only be as clean as possible, not necessarily sterile.

To apply a pressure bandage, open the bandage (gauze, cravat, or strip) and place the center of the bandage directly over the wound. Maintain a steady pull on the bandage to keep the dressing in place as you wrap the ends of it around the body part. Tie the bandage with the knot directly over the wound. Check the pulse point to make certain that there is still circulation of blood to the area. The object is to control bleeding, **not** to stop the flow of blood to the extremity. If the fingers or toes of the injured body part develop cyanosis, if the digits become very cold, or if a pulse cannot be found, the bandage should be loosened just enough to allow circulation to return to the area.

Tourniquet

A tourniquet is a device used to control bleeding that cannot be stopped by any combination of direct pressure, elevation, or pressure on the supplying artery. **A tourniquet is to be used only as a last resort** and only on the extremities (arms or legs). The decision to apply a tourniquet is, in reality, a decision to sacrifice a limb in order to save the individual's life. Once a tourniquet has been applied, physician care is imperative. Application of a tourniquet is rarely necessary and should be considered only when a large artery has been severely damaged and bleeding is profuse and out of control.

Internal Bleeding

Blunt trauma or pelvic fractures can result in internal bleeding. While this type of bleeding is not visible, it can result in serious damage, even death. The patient can go into shock before medical personnel are aware that there is bleeding.

Any time a patient has a fracture (particularly of the hip or pelvis), damage to the chest area, or a penetrating wound of the abdomen or skull, medical personnel should suspect internal bleeding.

Signs and Symptoms

Common signs and symptoms of internal bleeding include:

- Bruises.
- Pain, tenderness, swelling, or discoloration at the injury site.
- Bleeding from body orifices such as the mouth, rectum, and so on.
- Cold and clammy skin.
- Restlessness, combativeness, or anxiety.
- Dilated pupils.
- Thirst.
- Altered level of consciousness.
- Decreasing blood pressure.
- Nausea and vomiting.
- Increasing pulse rate.
- Rigid abdomen on palpation.
- Vomiting coffeeground-like substance (blood).

Emergency Treatment

1. Notify the physician.
2. Check for fractures.
3. Maintain an open airway. If ordered, administer oxygen.
4. Keep the patient quiet; loosen restrictive clothing. If no spinal injuries or fractures of the lower extremities are suspected, elevate the patient's feet.
5. Monitor vital signs every 3–4 minutes.
6. Assist the physician as necessary.
7. If physician is absent, activate EMS.

Wounds

Wounds are generally classified as closed and open. The general first aid for various wounds will be presented.

Closed Wounds

In this type of injury, there is no break in the continuity of the skin. The damage has occurred beneath the skin to the soft tissue. Closed wounds are characterized by swelling and pain at the injury site, redness or discoloration (called ecchymosis), and localized heat. Sometimes large vessels have been damaged, resulting in a collection of blood beneath the skin called a hematoma.

Emergency Treatment   Small bruises usually require no first-aid treatment. Larger bruises can be treated by applying ice or cold compresses to the injury site. Be sure to wrap up the ice or compress in a towel to avoid frostbite to the area. Apply the ice to the area for 20 minutes and then remove for 20 minutes. Applying ice relieves the pain and reduces swelling. Elevation of the affected limb may be indicated to help reduce pain and swelling.

At times, it is hard to detect if any internal bleeding is present. Office personnel should treat for internal bleeding if there is doubt. In addition, if there is a large bruised area, check for fracture.

Open Wounds

An opening or a break in the continuity of the skin can result in external hemorrhaging and wound contamination. An open wound may be an indication of a more serious problem, such as a fracture. Open wounds are classified according to cause and/or appearance and include lacerations, avulsions, punctures, abrasions, and incisions.

Lacerations   A laceration is a tear in the skin and underlying tissue that produces ragged edges. Lacerations can cause severe bleeding if a blood vessel is cut. Healing is difficult because of the jagged edges, which may have contaminated matter that can lead to infection. In addition, the edges of the skin may have torn or missing sections.

Emergency Treatment

1. Notify the physician.
2. Control bleeding. Use direct pressure, elevation, and pressure on the supplying artery if necessary.
3. Remove surface dirt and loose debris. It may be necessary to flush the wound with soapy, distilled water.
4. The physician should examine the wound and either treat or order treatment.
5. Bandage as directed.

6. Determine the date of the last tetanus shot. If over 5 years ago, the patient may need a booster.

Avulsions Avulsion wounds occur when the skin is partially or completely torn off. Bleeding is quite profuse and scarring can be extensive. Common avulsion areas are the fingers, toes, hands, legs, feet, nose, penis, and forearms. These wounds can be caused by lawnmowers, power tools, animals, and automobile accidents.

Emergency Treatment

1. Notify the physician.
2. Clean the wound with warm, soapy distilled water.
3. If there is a skin flap, return it to its normal position.
4. If necessary, control bleeding by direct pressure.
5. The physician will treat the patient as necessary. Be prepared to assist.
6. Bandage as directed.
7. Determine the date of the last tetanus shot. If over 5 years ago, the patient may need a booster.
8. Chart the treatment given.

If the body part has been amputated:

1. Rinse the body part in sterile saline.
2. Wrap the body part in moist, sterile gauze, seal it in a plastic bag, and transport on ice in another container.
3. Never submerge the plastic bag in ice. This may freeze the tissue.

Punctures A puncture is caused by a sharp object that pierces and penetrates the skin and underlying structures. It is often difficult to determine the seriousness of this type of wound. While the puncture may appear small, it may be deep, which poses a dangerous chance of infection. In addition, internal organs may have been damaged.

Bleeding is not a problem in this type of wound unless the injury site is located in the chest or abdomen. Be sure to assess for an exit wound.

Emergency Treatment

1. Notify the physician.
2. Assess the patient for shock and internal bleeding.
3. Allow the wound to bleed freely for a few minutes to help clear the injury site of bacteria.

4. Clean the area with soap and distilled water. Soak the puncture for about 10 minutes in warm water and an antimicrobial soap.
5. The physician will examine and treat the injury.
6. Bandage as directed.
7. Determine the date of the last tetanus shot. If over 5 years ago, the patient may need a booster.
8. Chart the treatment given.
9. Give the patient a list of signs and symptoms of infection to watch for.

Note: If the impaling object is still in the wound, do not attempt to remove it. Notify the physician immediately.

Abrasions   This wound is a superficial scraping or rubbing of the epidermis and part of the dermis. Bleeding is usually not severe; however, oozing may be present. Abrasions are very painful because nerve endings are involved. If an abrasion covers a large area of the body, the chance for infection is great.

Emergency Treatment

1. Notify the physician.
2. Cleaning the wound may consist of scrubbing the area to remove debris. Follow the physician's orders on how to clean this type of wound.
3. Determine the date of the last tetanus shot. If over 5 years ago, the patient may need a booster.
4. Chart the treatment given.

Incisions   An incision is a straight, even separation of the skin. Bleeding can be profuse; damage to tendons and nerves may be present. Knives, razor blades, and broken glass are common objects that can cause incised wounds. This type of wound heals better than lacerations because of the smooth edges of the wound.

Emergency Treatment

1. Notify the physician.
2. Assess the patient for shock.
3. Control bleeding by using direct pressure.
4. Assist the physician as necessary.
5. Bandage as directed.
6. Determine the date of the last tetanus shot. If over 5 years ago, the patient may need a booster.
7. Chart the treatment given.

Dressings and Bandages

The basic purpose of dressings and bandages are to:

- Control bleeding.
- Prevent contamination of the wound.
- Protect the wound.
- Keep the wound dry and clean.
- Immobilize the wound site.

Different Types of Dressings and Bandages

It is necessary to be able to differentiate between the dressing and the bandage. A dressing is a sterile covering for the wound; it is layered and has coarse mesh gauze. There are different types of wound dressings that the physician may order (see Figure 8-2). They include:

- Aseptic (sterile gauze).
- Moist dressing.
- Petroleum gauze (a sterile gauze that has been saturated with petroleum to prevent sticking to the wound).
- Occlusive dressing (creates an airtight seal around the wound).
- Compress (bulky sterile dressing that helps to stop and control bleeding).
- Packed dressing (medicated gauze strips packed into wound).

Common Mistakes in Bandaging

Bandages hold a dressing in place over the wound, secure a splint to an injured body part, provide support, and help to control hemorrhaging. A bandage needs to fit securely without constricting blood flow. The two most common mistakes in bandaging are that the bandage is either wrapped too tightly or too loosely.

Applying Dressings and Bandages

Dressing and bandaging a wound takes adaptability, creativity, and patience. Medical personnel need to keep the following guidelines in mind:

- Always wear gloves.
- Use sterile material for dressings unless it is an emergency and none are readily available.

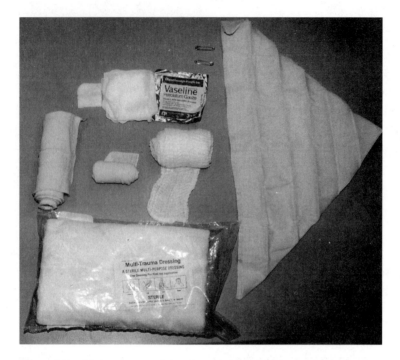

Figure 8-2   Various types of dressings and bandages.

- Open the dressing carefully and use sterile techniques to avoid contamination.
- The dressing should cover the wound completely.
- Anchor all bandages on first wind.
- Never bandage too tightly—the bandage should fit snugly.
- Avoid bandaging too loosely.
- The dressing should be completely covered by the bandage.
- Work from distal to proximal to reduce edema and congestion.
- Leave fingers and toes exposed to assess circulation.
- Always bandage the injured part in the position of function.
- Ask the patient if they feel any tingling or discomfort caused by the bandage.

Medical personnel should adapt the bandaging to the location of the injury or wound. Remember to follow the guidelines given to ensure a proper bandaging of the wound. There are a few additional applications that may be necessary in the physician's office.

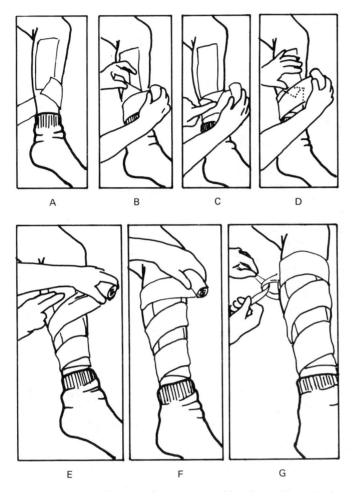

A B C D

E F G

Figure 8-3 Application of an open spiral bandage. (From Krebs and Wise, *Medical Assisting, Clinical Competencies,* © 1994, Delmar Publishers.)

Pressure Dressing Cover the wound with a bulky sterile dressing. Apply pressure, if necessary, until the bleeding stops. Using a firm roller bandage, apply the bandage over the dressing and secure it.

Spiral Bandage Secure the bandage. Wrap the roller gauze around the limb approximately 1/2 to 1/4 the width of the bandage. Continue until the dressing is covered by at least 1 in. on all sides, and secure the bandage with safety pins or tape, or tie the bandage off (see Figure 8-3).

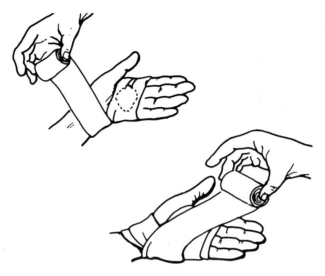

Figure 8-4   Figure-eight bandage. (From Krebs and Wise, *Medical Assisting, Clinical Competencies,* © 1994, Delmar Publishers.)

Figure-Eight Bandage   The figure-eight is used when bandaging a joint. The roller gauze should be secured by wrapping around the area below the joint. Turn the small corner of the end of the roll next to the skin over the first complete wrap. Continue to wind around the limb several times. Alternate wrapping below the joint and above the joint, covering the joint itself. This procedure allows the limb to bend without disturbing the bandage (see Figure 8-4).

Sling   Using a triangular bandage: Place one end of the base of the open triangular bandage over the shoulder of the uninjured side. Have the point of the triangular bandage on the injured side, with the point toward the injured elbow. Bring the loose end of the bandage up over the bent arm to the shoulder on the injured side. The entire hand must be supported, with finger tips exposed to access circulation. Be sure that the hand is elevated 15 degrees. Tie a knot at the neck on the uninjured side. Do not tie the knot over the spinal column at the back of the neck—the knot should be toward the side. Gauze pads may be placed under the knot to cushion it. Either pin or tie the loose end of the bandage at the elbow (see Figure 8-5). A cravat can be used as a chest binder to help keep the injured limb in place. Ask if the patient is comfortable. Assess the fingers for coldness, cyanosis, and sensation.

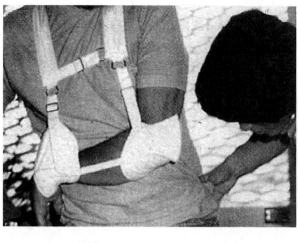

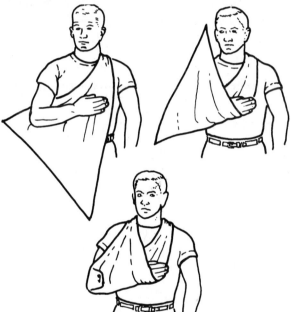

Figure 8-5 (a) Buckle type of arm sling for support. (b) Applying an arm sling (From Krebs and Wise, *Medical Assisting, Clinical Competencies,* © 1994, Delmar Publishers.)

Summary

Because it is possible for a patient to bleed to death within minutes, the medical office staff will need to respond to bleeding injuries without delay. Identifying the source of bleeding, taking action to control it, and properly treating the injury are skills that the health care professional needs to develop.

Review Questions

1. List 3 functions of blood and identify the element that is primarily responsible for the function.
2. Of the 3 types of bleeding, identify the most life-threatening and explain why.
3. List the physical characteristics of venous and arterial bleeding.
4. Why is hemophilia dangerous in a wound situation?
5. List the 5 steps in controlling bleeding, and the rationale for each.
6. Which artery would you use to help control bleeding in the thigh? Knee area? Forearm?
7. When is a pressure bandage appropriate, and how is it applied?

Chapter 9

Shock

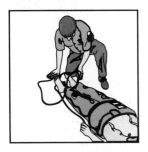

Objectives

After completing this chapter the learner should be able to:

1. Identify the changes that occur with individual body systems when an individual experiences shock.
2. List the different types of shock according to their causes.
3. Recognize the signs and symptoms of shock.
4. List the steps involved in treating shock and the rationale for each.

Introduction

When the circulatory system does not provide enough blood to all vital organs, the body reacts in a condition called shock. Shock is a life-threatening situation that can occur after serious injury, severe emotional trauma, or the sudden onset of illness. If left unchecked, the patient can die from shock alone. Medical personnel should always treat patients for shock because shock progresses in an irreversible step-by-step process. Therefore, the signs and symptoms must be recognized and appropriate measures taken to prevent or reduce the severity of shock.

Anatomical Overview

Whenever the body is damaged in any way, it will take steps to correct the problem. Often this effort will lead to more problems. In effect, a vicious cycle is established that can only harm or kill the patient. The basic problem begins with the circulatory system. Within this system, several different problems initially occur:

- The heart fails to pump enough blood or stops pumping altogether. This occurs with cardiac arrest or myocardial infarction.
- Blood escapes through torn or damaged blood vessels. This occurs with wounds.
- Blood volume decreases, caused by blood loss or dilation of blood vessels to a size that causes the blood pressure to drop. Psychogenic shock and syncope (fainting) are examples of this type of problem.

If there is decreased blood volume due to bleeding, often the body will make an effort to increase the blood flow to vital organs by increasing the pumping action of the heart. This will cause an increase in blood loss, resulting in a further decrease in blood volume, which leads to decreasing blood pressure. All of this useless action of the heart causes severe strain; eventually it will lead to heart failure and then to cardiac arrest, which in turn will cause death. Shock, once it progresses, is not reversible through any medical treatment. It can, however, be prevented or halted in its progression, breaking this vicious cycle and improving the patient's chances for survival.

Classifications of Shock

While the type of shock does not affect the basic treatment, further treatment may vary from one cause to the next. Classifications of shock are presented in Table 9-1.

Signs and Symptoms of Shock

Signs and symptoms of shock will vary from patient to patient. Knowing the basic signs and symptoms, however, could save a patient's life. Patients **may be:**

- Restless and fearful/combative.
- Weak.

Table 9-1   Classifications of Shock according to Cause

Type of Shock	Cause
Hemorrhagic shock	blood loss
Cardiogenic shock	heart failure
Neurogenic shock	nervous system failure
Anaphylactic shock	severe allergic reaction
Psychogenic shock	dilated blood vessels
Metabolic shock	loss of body fluid
Septic shock	infection in the blood stream
Respiratory shock	lung failure

- Nauseated.
- Thirsty.
- Dizzy.
- Breathing in a shallow, rapid manner.
- Pale, cool, clammy.
- Experiencing a weak and rapid pulse.
- Cyanotic around the lips, tongue, and ear lobes.
- Confused, unresponsive, disoriented, suddenly unconscious.

Remembering that shock is a step-by-step process will help to clarify in what order these many signs and symptoms can occur. If the heart rate increases, then the pulse rate increases. While it is common for the pulse to be rapid after a traumatic incident or injury, it should begin to slow after several minutes. Next, the breathing rate increases in an attempt to make more oxygen available to organs being deprived due to the decreasing blood circulation.

Oxygen deprivation is often first felt by the patient as nameless fear and restlessness. Some individuals will react violently to this feeling. This behavior may be the first indication of shock. Additionally, in order to supply the available limited oxygen to vital organs, the body will shunt blood away from the peripheral area, resulting in cyanosis of the lips, nails, and oral mucous membranes. The skin will appear pale and cool. The patient will experience thirst. This is the body's attempt to replace lost blood volume by increasing fluid intake. Weakness and nausea are caused by the lack of oxygen and decreased blood supply to the digestive organs. These symptoms will intensify until all organs are affected, including the brain, resulting in disorientation, confusion, decreased awareness, or coma. Respiratory arrest that leads to cardiac arrest is the final stage in the development of shock.

Emergency Treatment

Medical personnel must treat each victim of trauma for shock. It is possible to keep a patient from going into shock by doing the following:

1. The patient should lie down and rest.
2. Maintain an open airway. Do not allow the patient's head to tilt forward, as this can cause the tongue to block the airway.
3. Control all external bleeding.
4. Maintain the body temperature of the patient. This may require placing a blanket under and over the patient. Maintaining the body temperature helps to facilitate a more adequate blood flow and prevents loss of body heat.
5. If there is no indication of spinal injuries or fractures to the lower extremities, elevate the legs 8–12 inches above heart level. This will help to return blood to the heart and brain. (If elevating the legs is contraindicated, lay the patient flat on the back. Be aware, however, that this patient is at risk of choking or aspirating if vomiting occurs and the patient is not rolled onto the side with the head supported.)
6. Give the patient nothing by mouth (NPO). (The patient might vomit or, with severe injuries, may require surgery.)
7. Monitor the pulse, breathing, and blood pressure at least every 5 minutes.
8. Provide emotional support.
9. If there are standing orders, you can administer oxygen accordingly.

Summary

While it is not possible to reverse the shock process through emergency treatment, prompt action on the part of the medical personnel can prevent or minimize the damage of shock. Prevention is the only sure way to treat shock.

Review Questions

1. List 3 emergency situations where shock may be a threat to life.
2. Explain why shock occurs.
3. List the classifications of shock and identify 1 cause for each.
4. List the signs and symptoms of shock.
5. List the treatment for shock and give a rationale for each step.

CHAPTER 10

Anaphylactic Shock

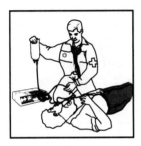

Objectives

After completing this chapter the learner should be able to:

1. Define anaphylactic shock and its most common cause.
2. Identify the physical changes that occur when an individual experiences anaphylactic shock.
3. Explain the effect of histamine, serotonin, and bradykinin on the body.
4. Identify the clinical features of life-threatening, as well as less severe, symptoms of anaphylactic shock.
5. Identify the basic steps in treating anaphylactic shock.
6. Recognize the necessity of developing individual protocols for dealing with anaphylactic shock.

Introduction

Anaphylactic shock is a severe allergic reaction to a specific substance. When it occurs, it is a life-threatening emergency. Death can occur within 15 minutes following a severe reaction. Medical personnel need to recognize and respond immediately to this dangerous situation.

Common Causes of Anaphylactic Shock

This type of severe allergic reaction occurs when the body comes into contact with an antigen that causes physiological changes. This reaction typically occurs less than 1 minute after exposure. The most common causes are parenteral medications, insect stings, and immunotherapy for allergies. Less commonly, the reaction occurs after a particular food or drug has been ingested. The faster the antigen enters the blood stream, the faster the reaction of the body.

The body, reacting as if it were being attacked by the antigen, sets in motion a chain of events that is intended for self-protection. In reality, however, the patient experiences physiological changes that could be fatal. Everyone who is involved in the dispersement of medication should be aware of the possibility of this severe reaction and be trained in the steps to counteract its effects on the body. As with other types of shock, prevention is the best treatment.

Prevention of Anaphylactic Shock

Patients should be questioned about allergies before receiving medications. Careful examination of the chart for documented allergies is a must. It should be stressed to **all** patients to call the office if they experience any difficulties after taking medication, both prescribed and OTC (over-the-counter). All complaints should be documented and referred to the physician for evaluation.

Known allergies should be stamped on the front of the patient's chart and on all pages inside, in red for greater visibility. Because severe allergic reactions can happen any time to anyone, it is not possible to predict when this type of shock will occur. Therefore, every precaution must be taken for those individuals who have already experienced any type of reaction to a substance. These individuals should be encouraged to wear Medic Alert tags and to carry an anaphylaxis kit if prescribed by the physician.

Physical Changes

Anaphylaxis can occur after a single exposure to an antigen, such as blood transfusions, or following repeated exposures, as is the case with medication. Within the immune system several changes occur. In response to the first antigenic stimulus, production of IgE antibodies takes place. These antibodies adhere to mast cells, which are found in connective tissue and contain slow-reacting substance (SRA), serotonin, bradykinin, and histamine. As the antigen attaches to the antibody, mast cells break down and release the chemicals mentioned above. Each chemical elicits a specific response from the body that causes the visible physical problems associated with anaphylactic shock. Histamine causes the dilation of the blood vessels and makes them susceptible to plasma leakage. The leakage of the plasma causes edema of the tissues, contraction of smooth muscle, and marked increase of capillary permeability. Serotonin causes peripheral blood vessel contraction (decreasing the blood return to the heart), contraction of smooth muscle, and increased capillary permeability. SRA causes severe bronchial constriction. Although its effects are delayed, the symptoms persist for hours. Bradykinin also reacts slowly. It greatly increases capillary permeability, releasing fluid into the tissues, causing edema, smooth-muscle contraction, and pain.

The pooling of blood caused by peripheral resistance and increased permeability of vessels reduces the blood return to the heart. Blood pressure begins to fall, effective tissue perfusion declines, and waste products collect within the blood and tissues. The end result of these effects can be respiratory and cardiac arrest if this situation is left unchecked.

Signs and Symptoms

The clinical features of anaphylaxis can be divided into two major categories:

Less Severe Symptoms Less severe symptoms include:

- Anxiety.
- Flushed and dry skin.
- Hives/itching.
- Edema of the lips and/or tongue.
- Cyanosis of the lips.
- Nasal congestion.
- Stomach cramping.
- Nausea.
- Diarrhea.
- Sudden sneezing.
- Rhinorrhea.

Life-Threatening Symptoms Life-threatening symptoms include:

- Weakness.
- Difficult and rapid breathing.
- Weak and rapid pulse—over 100.
- Hypotension.

- Shock.
- Cardiac irregularities.
- Restlessness, often followed by loss of consciousness.
- Acute respiratory failure.
- Acute cardiac failure.

While not every symptom will be present, the office personnel should always be alert for early detection of this type of shock.

Emergency Treatment

The steps in treating this situation must be quickly initiated and will require the presence of a physician. It is necessary that this type of emergency response be discussed and the responsibilities assigned before it occurs. The physician and staff must work together to develop a protocol that every member of the team is comfortable with. What will be given here are the steps necessary to administer emergency care quickly and efficiently. This protocol is not intended to represent the only way to deliver this type of care, but it is a basis on which discussion should revolve.

After noticing the start of clinical features of anaphylactic shock, the medical personnel should:

1. Bring the crash drawer to the patient. Table 10-1 lists the drugs, dosages, and equipment normally needed to treat anaphylactic shock.
2. Maintain an open airway.
3. Take vital signs—BP, pulse, respiration.
4. Call EMS.

Assess the patient's breathing. In the event of obstruction, give mouth-to-mouth resuscitation, or insert an oral airway and apply mechanical ventilation. If the patient is breathing but experiencing difficulty and there is a standing order, administer oxygen at 4 liters per minute via a mask. The patient should be in the semi-Fowler's position for best results.

Another member of the team should be taking vital signs, recording the information, and reporting this information to the physician, if not present. The administration of epinephrine is usually the most efficient treatment for anaphylactic shock. The recommended dosage is 0.2–1 ml epinephrine 1:1000 IM or subcutaneously. If needed, the dose may be repeated 4–5 times at 3–5 minute intervals. Be sure to vigorously massage the injection site to increase absorption. Additional treatment may include the administration of an antihistamine. The recommended dosage is 25–50 mg diphenhydramine (Benadryl) p.o., IM, or IV

Table 10-1   Crash Drawer

Drugs	Dosage	Equipment
A. Epinephrine, 1:1000 IM if IV: 1:10,000	1 ml q 3–5 minutes, maximum	1 ml syringe, 5/8–2 in. needles.
B. Benadryl	25–50 ml, IM or IV	Butterfly needle #19 & 21 Angiocath/if IM: 3 ml syringe 5/8–2 in. needle
C. aminophylline	5.6 mg/kg of body weight IV (usually 250–500 mg in 5% dextrose in water used in severe reactions to combat bronchospasm)	Tourniquet, alcohol preps, IV tubing Butterfly needle 19 & 21 Angiocath
D. Ringer's solution		
E. 5% dextrose in water		

depending upon the patient's age, weight, and condition. The physician may start to administer Ringer's solution through a large-bore catheter. The large-bore catheter makes it easier to give medications by IV. If the blood pressure continues to fall or drops rapidly, the use of a vasomotor drug (such as norepinephrine) to constrict blood vessels may be indicated. If injected, watch the injection site closely for signs of drug infiltration. Those signs include redness and swelling. Report this development to the physician immediately.

Because the need for action is immediate in this type of emergency, office personnel need to discuss their responsibilities and complete a practice drill in order to develop a smooth team response. The potential for this life-threatening situation occurs every time a patient takes a medication. There is an additional responsibility for medical office personnel when parenteral medication is administered. No patient should be allowed to leave the office until at least 20 minutes have passed since the injection was given. In addition, accurate documentation is essential concerning any problems patients may experience in taking medications.

Summary

Administering medications is a common occurrence in the medical office, and the majority of patients will have no adverse reaction. For those individuals who experience anaphylactic shock, a well-trained and prepared office staff can make the difference between life and death.

Review Questions

1. List the precautions that health care providers can take to prevent anaphylactic shock.
2. List the chemicals that are released in response to an antigen-antibody reaction.
3. Describe how each chemical affects the body.
4. Based on the effects of the chemicals in question #3, describe the patient's appearance.
5. List the treatment for anaphylactic shock.

CHAPTER 11

Sudden Illness

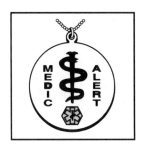

Objectives

After completing this chapter the learner should be able to:

1. Define syncope and its treatment.
2. Describe each stage of a tonic-clonic seizure.
3. List the treatment for a tonic-clonic seizure.
4. Define status epilepticus.
5. List the different causes of stroke.
6. Describe the common signs and symptoms of stroke.
7. List the medical office's responsibilities in treating the emergency stroke patient.
8. Define Diabetes Type I, Type II, and Gestational Diabetes.
9. Describe the signs and symptoms of diabetic coma and insulin shock.
10. Describe the appropriate treatment for diabetic coma and insulin shock.
11. List the correct steps to use in drawing up insulin.
12. Describe the function of insulin and glucose.
13. Explain the body's physiological response to cold.
14. Define hypothermia.

15. List four contributing factors to hypothermia.

16. Describe the emergency care that should be given to a patient with hypothermia.

17. Describe frostbite and the emergency treatment that should be given.

Introduction

Sudden illness, psychological or physical, can happen at any time. According to Miller-Keane's medical dictionary, illness is defined as "a condition marked by pronounced deviation from the normal, healthy state." This chapter will focus on sudden illnesses that are most commonly seen in a physician's office. Medical personnel are not to assume, however, that these are the only sudden illness situations that can arise.

Fainting

Syncope, or fainting, is a loss of consciousness that usually occurs when the brain is temporarily deprived of sufficient oxygen. This loss of consciousness is usually associated with severe pain, fright, unpleasant sights, hypoglycemia, certain drugs, cardiac arrhythmias, or other significant exposures that overwhelm the usual regulatory capacity of the nervous system.

Syncope occurs when there is sudden dilation of blood vessels, resulting in a decrease in the blood volume available for circulation. In addition, heart rate slows and blood pressure falls, further reducing the blood supply to the brain. Blood tends to pool in the dilated peripheral vessels, causing the individual to faint.

Signs and Symptoms

Fainting is not a disease in itself, but it may be the result of an underlying medical situation. Medical personnel must be able to recognize the signs and symptoms of fainting in order to handle the situation effectively. Fainting is most commonly preceded by:

- Nausea.
- Pallor.
- Sweating.
- Numbness.

- Tingling of the hands and feet.
- Cool, clammy skin.
- Lightheadedness.
- Seeing spots.
- Shakiness.

The individual may experience any of the identified symptoms, or immediate loss of consciousness may occur without any symptoms. Some individuals may experience signs to warn them of impending loss of consciousness. These warning signs may include:

- Weakness.
- Lightheadedness.
- Seeing spots.
- Nausea.
- Unsteadiness.

Emergency Treatment

If the individual has not fainted, but claims to feel faint, place the patient in a position that is appropriate for the circumstance. For example, when drawing blood, the patient is already seated. Place the head lower than the knees to improve circulation of blood to the brain. In most cases, this would be sufficient to prevent syncope from occurring. If the patient has difficulty breathing or has difficulty assuming this position, or if this position does not remedy the faint, place the patient on the back on the floor, with the feet elevated 8–12 in. **unless** the patient is suspected of having a cardiac condition. In this case, keep the patient lying flat so that the workload on the heart is not increased. In all cases, the patient is never left unattended and the physician is informed of the situation.

To care for an individual who has fainted:

1. Place the person in a supine position. Check for a medical alert necklace or bracelet.
2. Maintain an open airway. Check for life-threatening conditions and respond accordingly.
3. Elevate the feet 8–12 in. unless the person has a heart condition or back, neck, or leg injuries.
4. Administer spirits of ammonia. Break capsule and fan 6–8 in. below nose to avoid burning mucosa.
5. Loosen any tight clothing that might restrict free breathing.

6. Do not give anything to eat or drink unless the individual is **fully** conscious.

7. Wipe the patient's forehead with a cool, wet cloth. **Never** splash or throw water in the face of a patient. Water can be aspirated into the lungs and cause respiratory distress.

8. If the patient vomits, place the individual in the coma position (see Figure 11-1). Roll the patient onto a side, knees bent, the arm closest to the floor bent under the head for support; this allows vomitus and other fluids to drain from the mouth. The mouth should be gently wiped out with a soft cloth. Medical personnel must be certain that latex gloves are worn and that universal precautions are used in each instance.

Seizures

Seizures occur when electrical activity involved in normal brain cell functioning is interrupted, causing communication between the brain and the rest of the body to be temporarily ineffective. Seizures do not constitute a specific disease. They are a manifestation of various conditions causing over-stimulation of the brain's nerve cells. The most common condition causing seizure activity is epilepsy. Other causes include traumatic injury to the brain, infection, toxicity, and fever; seizures can be drug induced or idiopathic. For a more complete listing of seizure types and causes, see Seizure Response Guide in Chapter 3 beginning on page 42.

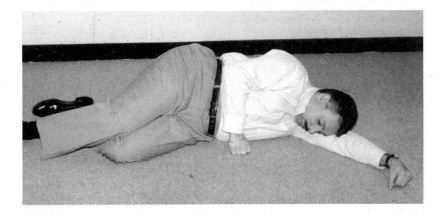

Figure 11-1 Coma Position.

While there are many different types of seizures, this chapter deals primarily with generalized tonic-clonic (grand mal) seizures and the condition known as status epilepticus.

Generalized tonic-clonic seizures occur when there is an interruption of electrical impulses in the brain cells. This disruption causes the characteristics that are associated with this type of seizure activity. Generalized tonic-clonic seizures can be very frightening for the individual witnessing the seizure as well as for the person experiencing it. Care must be taken to assist the patient as well as to reassure others in the immediate area.

Signs and Symptoms

Many times an individual will experience an aura before a seizure. An aura is an early warning sign that a generalized tonic-clonic seizure is about to occur. It usually lasts only a few seconds and involves particular sensations: hallucinations of sight and sound, experiencing an unpleasant smell, an unpleasant taste in the mouth, numbness in a specific body area, unpleasant sensation in the stomach that has been described as similar to a roller coaster ride, and tingling or twitching in a specific part of the body. In epilepsy this aura can serve as a warning that allows the patient to move to an area of safety before the seizure actually begins.

Phases of Tonic-Clonic Seizures

Generalized tonic-clonic seizures move through three stages: the tonic phase, the clonic phase, and the postictal phase.

Tonic Phase As the seizure begins (the tonic phase), there is a continuous contraction of all muscles, the eyes roll back, and the patient loses consciousness. This phase can last up to 30 seconds. During this time the body is completely rigid; breathing is compromised due to the sustained contraction of respiratory muscles. In some cases the patient may emit a high-pitched cry, the result of abdominal muscle contractions forcing air past the vocal cords. This cry is not an indication of pain. The patient may also experience increased salivation, dilated pupils, and pupils that are nonreactive to light.

Clonic Phase The patient then experiences the clonic phase of the seizure. During this phase the patient will have intermittent contractions and relaxation of the skeletal muscles, resulting in violent jerking movements of the arms and legs. It is during this phase, which can last from a few seconds to 3–5 minutes, that patients can seriously injure themselves. These forceful and intermittent contractions further compromise respiration. In some individuals apnea will occur, generally only lasting about a minute. An involuntary loss of bowel and bladder control is not uncommon during this phase, and some patients will appear to be frothing at the mouth through clenched jaws. As muscular contractions become less frequent and the periods of relaxation become longer, the clonic phase gradually comes to an end. The end of the clonic phase is typically signaled by a deep breath followed by shallow, irregular breathing.

Postictal Phase The postictal phase is the last phase of the seizure. This phase generally lasts 5–30 minutes, but can last several hours. During this phase the patient may be somewhat disoriented at first and may experience headache, drowsiness, and fatigue; the patient may not remember the seizure. Generalized tonic-clonic seizures usually last an average of 5 minutes.

Status Epilepticus

In the condition known as status epilepticus, this single seizure may last 5–10 minutes, or may be a series of seizures that occur in rapid succession and do not allow the patient to regain consciousness. This condition is a medical emergency. In half of the cases where it occurs, the result is death because of complications brought on or aggravated by the patient's medical status. Because of prolonged oxygen deprivation to the brain, irreversible brain damage can occur.

In order to effectively and safely assist an individual experiencing a seizure, it is important for medical personnel to know what actions may cause harm to the patient, as well as those techniques that would typically be the most helpful (see Table 11-1).

Emergency Treatment

If medical personnel have a padded tongue blade accessible before the patient's teeth become clenched, it can be inserted between the teeth to keep the patient from biting the tongue and causing bleeding into the mouth. During the seizure this blood could pool at the back of the throat, causing an airway obstruction and possible aspiration into the lungs.

The Medical Assistant or Allied Health Professional may insert a nasal airway if the physician has instituted a standing order for its insertion after seizure activity has stopped and if airway is blocked.

When the seizure subsides, care should be taken to protect the patient's physical and emotional status. Put the patient in the coma position and protect from any unnecessary movement. Remain with the patient to offer reassurance and assist in reorienting the individual. Continue to monitor breathing and other vital signs.

Table 11-1   DOs and DO NOTs for Seizures

Do	Do Not
1. Immediately alert the physician to the situation so a determination can be made as to emergency status.	1. **Do not** hold the patient down or restrict seizure activity. Holding a patient in seizure can break bones and cause soft tissue injury because of skeletal muscle rigidity.
2. Protect the patient from harm by removing any objects that might be in the way of the body movements of the patient. Cushion the patient's head with something soft to protect the head from hitting the floor and causing injury.	2. **Do not** force anything between the patient's clenched teeth. This can cause soft tissue injury to the mouth and damage or break teeth, which would fall back into the throat; if the patient is wearing dentures, pressure could loosen them and allow the dentures to fall to the back of the throat, causing an airway obstruction.
3. Maintain an open airway. The administration of high-concentration oxygen may be ordered by the physician and should be easily accessible.	
4. Obtain, record, and monitor vital signs.	
5. Loosen any tight clothing to reduce restriction of movement and respiration. Remove any eye-glasses.	
6. Cover the patient for warmth and to alleviate embarrassment to the patient once the seizure is over.	
7. Be cautious of what is said during the seizure. The patient may be able to hear what is going on in the immediate area.	
8. Preserve patient's dignity at all times.	

Status epilepticus presents a life-threatening situation for the patient, and additional treatment is required. This condition is characterized by continuous seizuring. It will be necessary for the medical professional to follow individual office protocol.

Stroke

Any process that impairs the circulation of the brain can result in a cerebrovascular accident (CVA), commonly called stroke. Stroke is the third most common cause of death in the United States. These incidents rise with age and are more commonly seen in males. Approximately half of all individuals who experience stroke will either die or suffer permanent neurological damage as a result. Rapid transport, proper treatment, and medical advances in treatment increase the patient's chances of recovery. Likely candidates for stroke include individuals with hypertension, a history of transient ischemic attacks (TIAs), diabetes, high cholesterol levels, sclerosis of carotid arteries or vessels of the heart, and gout.

Causes of Stroke

Causes of stroke include thrombosis, embolus, and aneurysm or hemorrhage.

Thrombosis   Thrombosis is the most common cause of stroke. It occurs when a cerebral artery is blocked by a clot that forms within the artery itself. Approximately 80 percent of all strokes are caused by thrombosis.

The condition of arteriosclerosis, in which plaque builds up inside the artery, is the major cause of the formation of the blood clot. As this plaque builds up along the arterial wall and narrows the passageway, blood flow is slowed considerably; the plaque deposits eventually cause clots. If the clots become large enough, they can cut off the blood flow to the artery, in turn reducing the blood flow to areas of the brain tissue. This tissue dies rapidly from lack of oxygen.

Transient Ischemic Attacks   Up to 2/3 of all strokes caused by thrombosis are preceded by transient ischemic attacks (TIAs). TIAs occur when the blockage is incomplete or lasts only a few minutes. A series of TIAs can occur over a period of time, usually getting worse with time. TIAs cause no permanent brain damage but may be a forewarning of a stroke.

Symptoms of TIAs usually last for less than 24 hours and commonly for less than 1 hour. Some common symptoms of TIAs include:

- Blindness in one eye.
- Dizziness.
- Headache.
- Fainting.
- Temporary paralysis of the face.
- Temporary paralysis of one side of the body.

- Inability to recognize familiar objects.
- Difficulty in pronouncing words.

Embolus An embolus is a blood clot or fatty substance such as fatty plaque that breaks loose and travels through the body via the bloodstream, becoming lodged in one of the cerebral arteries. This type of stroke has a rapid onset. Incidence is higher in young or middle-aged adults. It occurs frequently in individuals with existing heart disease.

Aneurysm Aneurysm causes stroke in 15–25 percent of patients. Hemorrhage occurs when a diseased blood vessel bursts in the brain, releasing blood into the brain tissue. About 80 percent of these individuals will experience rapid onset and death. Severe headache and vomiting are common symptoms. Incidents are higher among individuals suffering from hypertension and arteriosclerosis. Occurrence is at any age, but aging increases the chances of hemorrhage occurring.

Signs and Symptoms

No matter the cause, the signs and symptoms of stroke depend on the location, size, and severity of the stroke. However, the precise signs and symptoms that accompany the stroke are determined by the cause. Thrombosis stroke results in a lessening of bodily functions without pain; onset is gradual. Hemorrhagic stroke produces severe headache that results in a loss of consciousness. Embolic stroke is characterized by sudden convulsions, paralysis, and loss of consciousness.

General signs and symptoms are:

- Loss or impairment of motor function.
- Decreasing or altered level of consciousness.
- Difficulty in communication.
- Partial or total paralysis on one side.
- Visual and sensory changes.
- Headache.
- Respiratory distress.
- Pupils unequal.
- Loss of bowel or bladder control.

Emergency Treatment

It is important to note that emergency care is the same regardless of the cause. However, additional care and long-term care will be affected by the cause. Medical personnel will need to question family members who were present at the time the stroke occurred. A complete history from the family is invaluable in establishing continual care.

Immediate emergency care consists of activating EMS and notifying the physician immediately. If the patient is brought to the office, the following steps may be initiated, depending upon office protocol:

1. Handle patient carefully and calmly. Remember, even if unable to communicate, the patient can probably hear and understand what is said.

2. Position patient on back with head and shoulders raised slightly, to relieve intracranial pressure. If patient is unconscious, an oral or nasal airway may be needed.

3. Assess respirations. Dentures and dental bridges may need to be removed.

4. Take vital signs. Take both carotid and radial pulses.

5. If patient becomes unconscious and/or experiences increasing difficulty in breathing, turn the patient on a side, preferably with the paralyzed side down.

6. Check for contact lenses and remove if present. If eyelids are affected, it may be necessary to loosely tape them down to prevent the eyes from drying out.

7. Maintain patient's temperature.

8. Keep patient absolutely quiet and still.

Remember that although the patient may appear to not hear or understand what is being said, often that is not the case. Because further stress can aggravate and worsen the stroke, it is necessary to remain calm. It may be necessary to relate this information to the patient's family to ensure their cooperation. Seeing a loved one paralyzed and unable to respond can be very frightening for the family.

Diabetes

Diabetes is caused by the inability of the pancreas to produce sufficient insulin for the body's needs. Insulin is a hormone manufactured in the beta cells or the Islets of Langerhans in the pancreas. This hormone is responsible for the proper metabolism of carbohydrates. Insulin is necessary for the absorption of glucose, the primary source of energy for the body, into the cells for their energy needs, and into the fat cells and liver for storage as glycogen. Between the action of insulin and glycogen, the body maintains a relatively constant blood concentration of glucose after eating and between meals. In a condition known as diabetes mellitus, however, the pancreas fails to secrete enough insulin. Glucose remains in the blood stream, causing certain changes within the body. First, blood-level glucose increases and a severely depleted supply of glucose for the cells occurs. All cells are deprived. In an attempt to provide enough energy to the cells, the body will use proteins as fuel, which eventually robs the muscles and vital organs of these necessary building blocks, reducing muscle and organ mass. In addition, the kidneys start spilling sugar into the urine in an attempt to reduce the glucose level of the bloodstream. The kidneys must also eliminate a large amount of water with the sugar, causing two conditions: polyuria (excessive urination) and polydipsia (excessive thirst). These conditions increase the danger of dehydration because the cells are not receiving adequate nutrition. The individual will experience extreme hunger that cannot be satisfied. In some individuals, weight loss occurs. The lack of nutrition to the cells also results in fatigue, both physical and mental. Of all the organs affected by the lack of glucose, the brain is the most susceptible to harm because it cannot utilize protein for energy. An imbalance between glucose in the bloodstream and the insulin available can cause life-threatening situations to occur.

Three Types of Diabetes

There are three types of diabetes: Type I (insulin-dependent diabetes), Type II (non-insulin-dependent diabetes), and gestational diabetes. The differences are based on whether insulin is required as a routine part of treatment, age of onset, and the severity of the disease.

Type I—Insulin-Dependent Type I (insulin-dependent) diabetes is typically first seen in people ages 10–16. It has, however, first appeared in individuals up to the age of 35. It develops rapidly. The beta cells of the pancreas are destroyed and insulin production ceases almost completely. Because of an immune response by the body, it is believed that this destruction occurs following a viral infection. In addition, hereditary factors are being investigated. These patients must follow a carefully regulated diet. In addition, insulin extracted from pork or beef, or made from human DNA (Humulin), must be injected subcutaneously (SQ) at regular times throughout the day. A patient's intake of nutrients and insulin regimen are highly individualized and adjusted by the physician according to the patient's life style, amount of exercise, and the severity of the disease. The balance of diet and insulin is essential to maintain a normal status quo. Any situation that upsets this balance can cause serious complications. Some examples of these situations are illness, exercise, overeating, and undereating. Illness such as fever and infection can increase the body's insulin requirements. Exercise can increase glucose requirements. Diabetics must learn to adjust their food intake and insulin injections. Urine and blood must be tested routinely for glucose levels.

Type II—Non-insulin-Dependent Type II (non-insulin-dependent) diabetes develops gradually and usually occurs in people over the age of 40. Most often, it is found during a routine medical examination. Insulin is produced in insufficient quantities to meet the body's needs, especially when the patient is overweight. These individuals do not require routine insulin injections. Treatment can consist of diet alone, or diet and oral medication to stimulate the pancreas to secrete more insulin. Some Type II diabetics may eventually require insulin injections. These individuals will also need to test urine and glucose routinely.

Gestational Diabetes (GDM) Gestational diabetes develops during pregnancy as a result of glucose intolerance. Characteristics of GDM are increased blood sugar during pregnancy. This rise in sugar results from deficiency of insulin that usually disappears after delivery, but in some cases returns many years later. Treatment will consist of a high-protein diet, increased intake of calcium and iron, and insulin injections.

Complications of Diabetes

Whatever type of diabetes, the patient who does not get proper treatment or fails to follow the physician's prescribed treatment may eventually develop cardiovascular disease, renal disorders, nerve damage, vision loss or blindness, and death. More immediate complications that can occur are diabetic ketoacidosis (diabetic coma) and insulin shock (see Table 11-2).

Diabetic Ketoacidosis Diabetic ketoacidosis is the result of an increased blood glucose and the production of fatty acids due to inadequate cellular sugar levels. Thus, fatty acids are formed from the body using the stored fat as a source of fuel at an excessive rate. These fatty acids are oxidized in the liver, leading to the increased formation of ketone bodies. These bodies result in metabolic acidosis. As mentioned before, dehydration can occur due to an increase in the production of urine by the kidneys. This loss of fluid can lead to hypotension.

Signs and Symptoms The patient experiences the following signs and symptoms of diabetic ketoacidosis:

- Kussmaul respirations (labored respiration and exaggerated air hunger caused by the body attempting to blow off carbon dioxide).
- Fruity odor on the breath (caused by fatty acids being converted to acetone and being expired in the air).

Table 11-2   Causes and Symptoms of Diabetic Coma and Insulin Shock

Diabetic Coma or Acidosis		Insulin Shock or Reaction	
Causes—Too little insulin, too much to eat, infections, fever, emotional stress.		Causes—Too much insulin or oral hypoglycemic drug, too little to eat, an unusual amount of exercise.	
Symptoms	Skin: Dry and flushed Behavior: Drowsy Mouth: Dry Thirst: Intense Hunger: Absent Vomiting: Common Respiration: Exaggerated, air-hungry Breath: Fruity odor of acetone Pulse: Weak and rapid Vision: Dim First Aid: Keep patient warm	Symptoms	Skin: Moist and pale Behavior: Often excited Mouth: Drooling Thirst: Absent Hunger: Present Vomiting: Usually absent Respiration: Normal or shallow Breath: Usually normal Pulse: Full and pounding (gives patient feeling of heart pounding) Vision: Diplopia (double) First aid: If conscious, give patient sugar or any food containing sugar (fruit juice, candy, crackers, etc.)
Obtain medical help immediately.		Obtain medical help immediately.	

Adapted from Keir, Wise and Krebs, *Medical Assisting, Administrative and Clinical Competencies*, Third edition, © 1993, Delmar Publishers.

- Decreasing levels of consciousness (caused by the inability of the brain to utilize any other sources of fuel).
- Frequent and severe abdominal pain (caused by fluid loss).
- Frequent urination (caused by the kidneys attempting to remove excess sugar).
- Irritability.
- Intense thirst (the body is attempting to replace lost fluid).
- Rapid, weak pulse.
- Flushed, dry, warm skin (loss of fluid).

The onset of diabetic coma develops in most cases over a 12–48 hour period. The patient grows progressively weaker and, without treatment, the patient will die.

Emergency Treatment Emergency treatment of diabetic ketoacidosis consists of:

1. Notifying the physician immediately.
2. Activating the EMS system.
3. Monitoring vital systems every few minutes. Be alert to additional symptoms of heart attack, stroke, or other cardiac problems as the cause of the coma.
4. Maintaining an open airway.
5. Being alert for vomiting. Have a suction machine available.
6. Treating the patient for shock.
7. Being prepared to administer insulin, if ordered by the physician.

Insulin Shock The other complication is insulin shock, occurring when there is too much insulin in the body, causing glucose to leave the bloodstream rapidly. Insulin shock occurs from the over-treatment of diabetes. The brain needs glucose as much as it needs oxygen to function, so it is the first organ to react to low blood glucose. Permanent brain damage or death can result if immediate action is not taken. Insulin shock has a rapid onset and is more often seen in children, due to their fluctuating dietary needs. Causes of insulin shock include any situation that causes an imbalance between dietary intake and the insulin administered. Increased exercise levels, severe emotional excitement, or exposure to severe cold also contributes to shock. Onset is very rapid, usually 5–20 minutes after the injection of too much insulin. Death can occur within minutes.

Signs and Symptoms Signs and symptoms of insulin shock include:

- Moist, pale skin.
- Hunger.
- Shallow breathing.
- Visual disturbances.
- Dizziness.
- Decreased level of consciousness.
- Speech difficulties.
- Tingling and numbness in the extremities.
- Confusion, anxiety, and combativeness.
- Profuse sweating.
- Convulsions in later stages.

Emergency Treatment Treatment of insulin shock consists of giving candy or a drink that contains sugar, if the patient is fully conscious. If the patient is semi-conscious, be sure the gag reflex is present. Test for this reflex by stimulating the patient's posterior pharynx with a tongue blade. If the patient does not respond, other treatment is necessary. The physician can administer (or leave a standing order to administer) Glucagon IM. A dose of 1 mg of Glucagon will increase blood sugar within 8–10 minutes. The medical personnel will see a response within 5–20 minutes.

Additional Supportive Care There are a few groups that will not respond with this treatment. They are very young children, alcoholics, and malnourished individuals. Additional supportive care includes:

- Maintaining an open airway.
- Administering of high-concentration oxygen (if ordered by the physician).
- Obtaining and recording all vital signs including the determination of a patient's level of consciousness.
- Maintaining body temperature.

Often it is impossible to differentiate between insulin shock and diabetic coma if the patient is unable to communicate.

Treatment for Undefined Diabetic Emergencies If medical personnel are doubtful whether the patient is suffering from too much or too little sugar in the bloodstream, administer sugar. If the patient is suffering from too little sugar, there will be an immediate positive response. When patients are suffering from too much sugar, their condition will probably not be worsened by this treatment. It is important to remember that insulin shock is a more immediate critical situation and can be treated successfully in the office.

If the condition indicates the administration of insulin, and the physician orders the injection, medical personnel need to be able to correctly draw up the prescribed amount and administer the injection properly.

Insulin

Insulin is a hormone secreted by the pancreas. It functions to enhance the transport of glucose into the cell, promote the synthesis of protein from amino acids, inhibit the breakdown of fat, and promote the synthesis of protein from amino acid. It has a very short half life of 3–4 minutes. Insulin supplements have been used since 1922. Insulin preparations are produced by pig or cow pancreas or by genetic engineering (Humulin). Short, intermediate, and long-acting preparations are available. Insulin must be injected because the acid of the stomach destroys its effectiveness. Injection is subcutaneous, and rotated body sites are used. In an emergency situation the upper arm and abdomen are easy-to-reach sites for administration (see Figures 11-2 and 11-3). Insulin is refrigerated and is given by a special syringe unit. Following the physician's order, office personnel will gently roll the vial between the palms. Do not shake the vial as the insulin will foam. Draw up the prescribed amount and, after cleaning the injection site with alcohol, insert the needle at a 90 degree angle; draw back the plunger to be sure that the needle is not in a blood vessel, and inject medication at a smooth, steady rate. The medical professional should activate the EMS as soon as possible. This patient will require further medical treatment. All injections should only be administered with a physician's order.

The medical personnel need to be familiar with the signs and symptoms of diabetic coma and insulin shock. The office staff may be responsible for defining these conditions to the newly diagnosed patient and family. Treatment protocol, once established by the office, should be reviewed and practiced. It may be necessary to instruct the patient and family in how to deal with these potential complications. While this type of emergency is rarely seen in the medical office, the potential for dealing with it through the patient and/or family is there. Certainly, this patient requires a great deal of educating by the medical office professional.

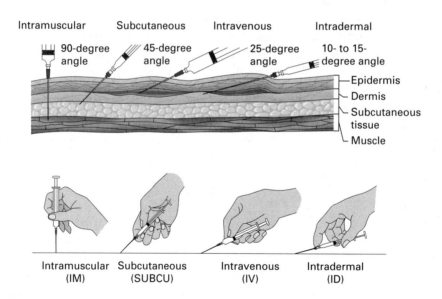

Figure 11-2 Angle of injections.

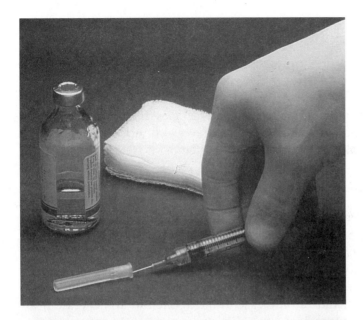

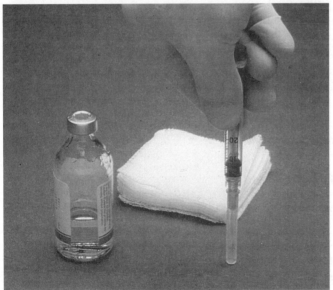

Figure 11-3 (a) Keeping one hand behind your back, "scoop" the cap onto the needle carefully so it does not become contaminated. (b) Secure the cap onto the hub of the syringe by pressing the tip against a hard surface. (From Krebs and Wise, *Medical Assisting, Clinical Competencies*, ©1994, Delmar Publishers.

Cold Emergencies

Exposure to cold temperatures can cause local injuries such as frostbite and frostnip. In some cases, it can lower the core body temperature to a degree where hypothermia and death can result. The temperature and length of exposure time are important contributors to cold emergencies. In addition, pediatric and geriatric patients, and patients in poor health or with serious health conditions, are more susceptible to the dangers of low temperatures.

Body's Normal Response to Cold

Normally, the body generates enough heat to maintain sufficient body temperature to maintain normal functioning. When faced with cold, the body must make certain physiological adjustments to maintain its core body temperature and to protect peripheral tissue.

First, the body increases its heat production and decreases its heat loss. Early responses to cold include an increase in metabolic rate to generate heat, and vasoconstriction to reduce heat loss.

Next, shivering occurs. Shivering is an involuntary contraction of muscles, which increases available body heat. Shivering occurs if the body temperature drops to below 95° F. However, shivering requires a great deal of energy by the body. Certain individuals, such as malnourished persons and diabetics experiencing insulin shock, will deplete their energy stores quickly and are more susceptible to the cold environment. Phenothiazines, barbiturates, and alcohol suppress or inhibit shivering in some individuals. Once shivering stops, body temperature can drop rapidly.

Signs and Symptoms of Hypothermia

The central nervous system becomes affected if core body temperature drops below 92°. Confusion, slurred speech, and amnesia can occur. The skin is cold and waxy; the face is pale and puffy. Heart rate begins to slow as metabolic needs drop because of the cold. As the temperature continues to drop below 90°, pupils become dilated; respiration slows; and hypotension, stupor, or coma occurs. At below 86°, pupils become fixed; coma, flaccid muscles, slow respiration, and possible cardiac arrest can occur. Below 82°, cyanosis, no spontaneous movement, unresponsiveness, barely detectable vital signs, slow irregular pulse, and cardiac arrest may occur.

It is possible to measure the body temperature with a specialized thermometer. Without this thermometer, however, office personnel will need to rely on the signs and symptoms described above to determine the level of hypothermia.

Contributing Factors to Hypothermia Contributing factors to hypothermia include:

- Age—Babies, children, and the elderly are most susceptible to cold.
- Long exposure—An environment that does not provide sufficient heat to maintain core body temperature will result over a long period of time in hypothermia. An example would be a house that is heated insufficiently.
- Trauma—Extreme blood loss can result in hypothermia, as can head, neck, and spinal injuries that disturb the body's thermoregulatory system. Near drownings can also result in hypothermia.
- Immobility—A patient who cannot move sufficiently to generate body heat may suffer from hypothermia.

Emergency Treatment of Hypothermia

Emergency treatment of hypothermia will depend upon the time it takes to transport the patient, and the degree of hypothermia. There are general guidelines that need to be followed regardless of the level of hypothermia the patient is experiencing. These guidelines are as follows:

1. Call the physician and/or EMS.
2. Avoid further heat loss. If clothing is wet, replace it with dry clothing or a blanket. Protect the patient from the wind.
3. If the respiratory rate and pulse are severely depressed, supplemental oxygen (with a physician's order) should be given at 50 percent. Be careful not to hyperventilate the patient as this can result in rapid change of the acidity of the blood and lead to arrhythmias. Airway devices may also be necessary.
4. Active rewarming should only be initiated in the hospital setting. The office can, however, administer humidified oxygen and **apply local heat** to large superficial blood vessels. Sugar water may be given to the patient who is conscious and capable of swallowing. (Do not administer alcoholic beverages, as they lower the core body temperature.)
5. Handle the patient gently.
6. Recognize that hypothermia can require up to 3–4 hours of CPR effort. The American Heart Association recommends that CPR be initiated on individuals where CPR would not ordinarily be started, such as in the

presence of fixed and dilated pupils. Be certain that there is no pulse before beginning CPR. A severe hypothermic patient will only breathe 3–4 times a minute and have a heartbeat of only 3–4 beats per minute.

External Cold Injuries

Frostbite is the literal freezing of body tissue, which often accompanies hypothermia. Frostbite most often affects the hands, feet, ears, cheeks, and nose. With continued exposure, this type of injury will progress from superficial to deep.

Within the body, the vasoconstriction that occurs to reduce heat loss leaves less heat to warm the superficial parts of the body. Ice crystals form between the cells, and the vasoconstriction worsens because of obstructed blood flow caused by the crystals. If left unchecked, deeper freezing of tissue occurs as water is extracted from cells and freezes. These ice crystals can cause cellular structural damage. Never massage or rub frostbitten parts because the movement of ice crystals can cause additional damage to the cells. In many cases, however, recovery is possible following proper rewarming.

Upon rewarming, significant vasodilation occurs in the area, resulting in a marked, flushed coloring. Swelling occurs due to capillary leakage. A mottled appearance may be present due to thrombosis in small vessels that affect circulation.

Factors that increase the likelihood of frostbite are trauma, age, tight or tightly-laced footwear, use of alcohol, wet clothing, use of nicotine, and race. Dark-skinned individuals are more likely to become frostbitten than any other race.

Three Stages of Frostbite

Medical personnel should recognize the three stages of frostbite; treatment differs according to the seriousness and degree of progress from stage to stage.

Stage 1—Frostnip Frostnip involves only the tip of the ears, nose, cheeks, fingers, toes, or chin. It is completely reversible. The patient is often unaware of the process because of loss of feeling. The first indication is a blanching of the skin. First aid consists of applying firm pressure with a hand or other body part (i.e., tucking fingers under the armpit) or blowing warm breath on the area. Upon rewarming, the area may be red, and a tingling sensation may be noted.

Stage 2—Superficial Frostbite If left unchecked, frostnip will develop into superficial frostbite, which is the freezing of water within the upper layers of the skin. The skin appears white, waxy, and firm, with the tissue below soft.

After thawing, the skin appears mottled with patchy, red-purple, and blanched areas. Edema and blisters that appear within 1–24 hours are usual. The affected area will tingle and be painful.

Stage 3—Deep Frostbite Deep frostbite occurs when the tissue beneath the skin is frozen solid to the touch. The skin is white to grayish blue and mottled. It is difficult to tell how deep the tissue is frozen. After thawing, the area may appear mottled and blue or gray.

Emergency Treatment of Frostbite

1. Never thaw the area if there is a chance of refreezing. Thawing is best done in a hospital setting if possible. Call EMS and/or physician.
2. Dress the injured area appropriately and transport.
3. If the area has been thawed, do not break any blisters that have formed. Cover the area with a sterile dressing after the physician's examination. Be sure to separate injured fingers and toes with small folded dressings.
4. Handle the area with care and do not allow the patient to walk on affected lower extremities.
5. Administer oxygen at the physician's direction.
6. Monitor vital signs.

Summary

Illness can occur suddenly and without warning. Often patients and their families not only seek treatment, but an explanation for why the illness occurred. The medical office staff will need to offer physical and emotional support to patients and their families.

Review Questions

1. Describe how treatment for syncope varies with individual patients.
2. Explain the stages of a tonic-clonic seizure.
3. You have a patient in the reception area who suddenly keels over and starts to twitch. Describe what you would do.
4. Describe how each cause of stroke can occur and the common signs and symptoms of each.
5. List the special needs that a stroke patient will have.

6. Describe the difference between TIAs and strokes.
7. Differentiate between hypoglycemia and insulin shock.
8. What are the major differences between Type I and Type II diabetes?
9. Explain the emergency treatment for diabetic ketoacidosis.
10. Define insulin, how it works, and when it is prescribed.
11. Explain how the body responds to cold.
12. What are the differences between hypothermia and frostbite?
13. Describe the three stages of frostbite.
14. Explain the emergency treatment for frostbite.

CHAPTER 12

Stress and Burnout

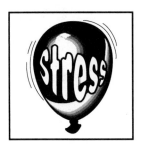

Objectives

After completing this chapter the learner should be able to:

1. Differentiate between stress and burnout, and between distress and eustress.

2. Identify and describe the four major causes of stress.

3. Define the fight-or-flight response and identify the physical changes that occur during this stress response.

4. Identify the physical, emotional, and social/behavioral signs and symptoms of stress.

5. Describe the nonproductive techniques typically used for coping with stress.

6. List productive and healthy methods for coping with stress/burnout.

7. Describe the factors that influence burnout.

8. Identify the characteristics of health care providers that are most at risk for burnout.

9. Identify the physical, emotional, and behavioral signs and symptoms of burnout.

10. Describe the techniques that the professional can implement to reduce the risk of burnout.

Introduction

Stewart Wolf once said, "An oyster's response to stress is to create a pearl." Unfortunately, in stressful situations, the human being's response is frequently the opposite—to intensify the situation by becoming increasingly negative. Most people must deal with stress on a regular basis. The best we can do is understand stress, recognize what causes it, and determine how to deal with it effectively on an individual basis.

Distress/Eustress

There are two types of stress—distress and eustress. Hans Selye, a major researcher in the field of stress and the discoverer of the General Adaptation Syndrome (GAS), defines distress as negative stress. It is damaging or unpleasant. The typical reactions associated with distress are anxiety, fear, worry, or agitation. Eustress is positive stress. It is pleasurable and satisfying. Eustress tends to heighten an individual's awareness, increase mental alertness, and contribute to increased cognitive and behavioral performance. When we hear the term "stress" used, however, it is usually taken to mean distress; the fact that eustress is also necessary to function effectively is seldom considered.

People generally perform best when they are under at least a mild to moderate amount of stress; too little stress is just as bad as too much. The goal of stress management is not to eliminate stress entirely, but to control it so that its effect is as motivating and productive as possible.

Causes of Stress

Most stress is caused by the way we think about and interpret the events that take place around us. An event that may cause serious distress for one individual may not affect someone else nearly as strongly. Some distress is real pressure caused by time demands, extraordinary life or work requirements, or danger. Other distress can be caused simply by worrying, particularly about situations where the individual has little or no control to alleviate stressful feelings.

The Four Major Sources of Stress

Stress can come from many places in our complex lives, but there are four major sources of stress. Recognizing these sources is the beginning of alleviating the stresses they cause.

Change Some people adapt easily to minor changes in their routine, lifestyle, or environment. Others become very upset and have difficulty coping or adjusting. Change can be minor—the rearrangement of a room, or a slight adjustment in time scheduling—or major—dealing with a serious illness, move, change in job, or adjustment in a relationship. Change is the most significant cause of distress for the population in general. For many medical professionals, a varied work routine is preferable—at a manageable pace. In an environment that is fast-paced most of the time, the professional needs to "take a breather," or periodic time-out, in order to stay consistently effective.

Absence of Approval Most individuals look to a variety of other people for approval of their actions, ideas, and personalities. Other people help to validate our feelings of societal worth, and help to influence an acceptable level of self-esteem. When that approval is not forthcoming, an individual's distress level tends to adjust inversely to the level of self-esteem at that point: low self-esteem, high stress.

Hopelessness At some point in the lives of most people, frequently as a result of a life crisis or major stressors, a feeling of hopelessness overwhelms them. For many this period of hopelessness is short-lived; for others, often because of life circumstances, the feeling persists. When people see no way out or no opportunity to achieve what they want from life, their stress level rises.

Increase in Hostility If you have ever watched two people argue, or have been involved in an argument yourself, you may recognize that certain changes took place. The situation may have started out as a conversation aimed at dealing with a specific problem. One person's voice may rise in order to make a point. The second person's voice rises to compensate and be heard. Before long, the individuals involved are shouting at each other. No one is listening because each is simply trying to be heard, and constructive interaction has come to a standstill. In fact, because people say things when they are angry that they normally wouldn't, the constructive intent of this situation may have taken several steps backward; regaining the potential working interaction may be difficult.

You may also notice that the participants become red-faced, more animated, and more intent on their task. A rise in anger or hostility for any reason increases an individual's stress level. Reactions show up in physical as well as emotional responses.

Physical Reactions to Stress

When an individual is experiencing stress, major body systems are affected, resulting in both visible and internal physical reactions. The systems primarily affected are the nervous, respiratory, endocrine, immune, cardiovascular, and digestive systems.

Physiological Responses

The effect of stress on the nervous system involves the emergence of what is known as the fight-or-flight reaction. The sympathetic nervous system exhibits this reaction and presents itself in the following responses:

- Increased blood pressure.
- Increased breathing rate. Anxiety hyperventilation can occur when the person is under extreme stress. Excessive ventilation of the blood supply as the blood attempts to release carbon dioxide causes light-headedness, dizziness, shortness of breath, and a pounding heart. The individual may also experience parathesia, a numbness or tingling in parts of the body; these signs are sometimes seen as signs of heart attack and can heighten anxiety.
- Increased mental activity and alertness.
- Increased sensory response.
- Increased energy release and strength in the muscles. The muscles tense, set, and get ready for action—either to take a stand and fight, or to flee.
- Blood flow to large active muscles increases, while there is decreased blood flow to the internal organs that are not needed for rapid activity such as the digestive organs.

Prolonged stress can contribute to high blood pressure, heart disease, and the development of ulcers.

Almost any kind of stress, whether physical or psychological, will lead to an almost immediate increase in the release of hormones from the adrenal glands. Hormones released include cortisol, epinephrine, and norepinephrine. Cortisol, also known as hydrocortisone, provides more energy to the body by converting the body's energy stores into glucose, a form of energy that the body can easily use. Cortisol, however, has also been linked to the suppression of the immune system, so that an individual's resistance to disease is lowered.

Epinephrine (adrenalin) and norepinephrine (nor-adrenalin) generally affect the body in the same manner as the sympathetic nervous system, by increasing the rate and strength of heart contractions and raising blood pressure. Epinephrine is fast-acting; it gets out of the blood stream quickly and seems to be released as a reaction to fear. Norepinephrine clears the blood stream more slowly and appears to be related to anger.

Physical and psychological stress can also change an individual's metabolism rate, influencing a person's mood, energy level, nervous irritability, and mental alertness.

When an individual is under extreme or prolonged stress, the immune system is negatively affected. Immunity is defined as "the ability of an individual to resist or overcome the effects of a particular disease or harmful agent." Allergies, including hay fever, urticaria, and asthma can develop or their reactions can become intensified. The immune system, at least for a period of time, is not functioning at its optimal level.

The cardiovascular system also responds to stress in unhealthy ways. Essential (common) hypertension comprises 90 percent of the cases of hypertension diagnosed, and can occur as a result of many things, yet nothing specific. Secondary hypertension is the result of a known disease process or specific medications and makes up the other 10 percent of all cases of hypertension. Examples of diseases that cause secondary hypertension include kidney disease and arteriosclerosis of the renal arteries.

Individual Reactions to Stress

While initial body systems react to stress or stressors in much the same way, an individual's personal reactions are unique. The individual's attitude and mind set influence how a situation is dealt with. A positive attitude is necessary to generate a productive resolution to a negative situation. It gives the individual personal control and action, as opposed to reaction, where personal control is unconsciously given up. Negative emotions such as anger, rage, hostility, distrust, and depression all affect an individual's health in a negative manner.

Experiencing all emotions, including negative emotions, is normal. Emotions are natural reactions to various circumstances, situations, and people. How we channel frequently generated emotional energy makes a big difference in whether we handle situations productively or negatively. If handled without tact, negative emotions can cause more damage than the situation that caused them.

A variety of individual reactions manifest themselves when people have to deal with stress. The health care provider is susceptible to these reactions and so is the patient, with the added illness or injury that brought the two together in the professional environment.

Behavioral Indicators

These reactions to stress vary in intensity and include the behavioral indicators in Table 12-1.

There are other reactions of a more individual nature. While everyone does not experience all of these signs and symptoms, most people can relate to at least a few of them.

Table 12-1   Behavioral Indicators of Stress

- Eating disorders.
- Grinding the teeth, especially while asleep.
- Sleep problems—insomnia, nightmares, inability to fall asleep.
- Muscle tension, particularly in the neck and shoulders.
- Frequent minor illnesses, such as colds.
- Indigestion/heartburn.
- Chronic fatigue.
- Frequent or persistent infections/cold sores.
- Increased alcohol or other drug use.
- Increased smoking.
- Depression/apathy/lethargy.
- Severe menstrual cramps.
- Inability to concentrate/indecisiveness/forgetfulness.
- Sexual dysfunction.
- Irrational or impulsive behavior.
- Irritability/anxiety.
- General feeling of weakness.
- Abdominal cramps/nausea.
- Diarrhea.
- Constipation.
- Shortness of breath/feeling faint/dizziness.
- Excessive sweating/clammy hands.
- Panic/fear.

Burnout

Everyone, regardless of the work that they do, is susceptible to stress (most notably distress) and experiences its physical as well as emotional effects until the stressful situation is resolved. While stress is viewed as the physical and emotional reaction of an individual to demands or damaging intrusion, burnout is reaction to prolonged stress in the extreme.

To "burn out" means "to fail, wear out, or become exhausted by making excessive demands on physical and/or emotional energy, strength, or resources." Burnout frequently occurs as a reaction to job-related stressors; individuals in the helping professions are particularly vulnerable. The physical demands of the job, as well as the varied emotional needs of patients (and sometimes co-workers), can take their toll on the health care provider's personal health unless burnout is recognized, understood, and dealt with productively and effectively.

Burnout and the Health Care Professional

Many who enter the helping professions do so out of a sincere desire to help others. The idealistic expectations of health care providers are often frustrated. First, there are situations where, no matter how skilled the provider, every patient cannot be returned to an excellent state of health. Also, in providing health care, it is often difficult to measure accomplishment or progress. Some conditions take a long time to improve, and frequently the only way some health care providers can keep track of how a patient is doing is by the written chart. Day-to-day or week-to-week progress cannot be seen face-to-face with each patient, especially in a large practice.

Working hours for health care professionals are frequently long. For the dedicated provider, the work goes on in the form of administrative duties, "on-call" status after regular office hours, or long consecutive hours. Realistically, if long hours are coupled with low pay, the professional health care provider may become frustrated. While those individuals at the highest levels of the helping professions may be well paid, paraprofessionals may be less satisfied with their salaries. When added to other job stressors, the individual may decide that it just is not worth it.

By the very nature of the varied helping professions, those most in need of care are frequently the least capable of expressing appreciation for the health care provider's attention and skillful assistance. Some patients (and their families) may feel that "this is what you get paid for" and may express those sentiments. Without positive or appreciative feedback, many health care providers feel unappreciated, and the quality of the care that they provide may start to deteriorate. The feeling is often, "If the patient doesn't care, then why should I?"

The health care professions cover so many aspects of an individual's well-being that it is common for providers to be thrown into situations for which they have been inadequately prepared. A medical assistant, for example, may be trained in administrative and clinical skills, but when faced with a violent or suicidal patient may be uncertain as to how the situation should best be handled.

In some areas of health care, professionals may be overloaded from lack of persons trained in the area, financial cutbacks, or lack of funding. The size of the facility may be small enough so that any overload comes in spurts, or other staff may call in sick. Being overloaded often means being overwhelmed by the workload.

The helping professions are difficult. In some health care areas it is common for patients or clients to be uncooperative and nonverbal due to mental illness, alcohol and/or other drug abuse, developmental delay, fear, or misunderstanding of the services that the professional is attempting to provide. No matter what the reason behind the behavior, it makes providing care more difficult.

In some health care professions, working conditions can be poor, unpleasant, or uncomfortable. There may be personality conflicts, lack of cooperation on the job, or differences in work and interaction style. For those going out into the community in public health service, the provider may come up against situations and environments that are physically and emotionally unhealthy.

At some point, many health care professionals realize that the system is not geared toward meeting the needs of everyone, and time for the highest quality of care is not always available. Public health clinics may have a substantial number of patients each day; it may seem like the facility is an assembly-line operation, with little time for individual patient/provider interaction. All facilities cannot help all patients, and facilities with a large number of patients may choose the quickest, generally most effective, and least expensive method of treatment without considering what is best for the individual patient.

Feelings of powerlessness can also be a significant factor in burnout. All of the patient education, communication, and appropriate feedback cannot assure that patients will follow those instructions in safeguarding or increasing their level of health. The health care provider cannot force anyone to comply with recommended treatment or lifestyle changes, no matter how simple or straightforward the situation or circumstances may be.

Reality often conflicts with the ideal academic training that the provider may have obtained. Every situation, every patient, every environment cannot be anticipated. Especially a new person in the field may have difficulty meshing reality with more idealistic expectations, aspirations, and training.

Some health care providers may find themselves in positions where the possibility for advancement is small or nonexistent. They may also find it difficult to acquire additional training without making a significant financial sacrifice, such as leaving their current position. These individuals may feel trapped, while others may be completely satisfied with the same position throughout their career.

Everyone runs the risk of professional/personal burnout unless symptoms are recognized and the situation is handled appropriately. Many excellent professionals leave their chosen fields each year because burnout became the overwhelming force in their professional persona. The time to handle burnout is before it begins, which means frequent personal evaluation.

Characteristics of Individuals Most at Risk for Burnout

Any professional who has a true need to give or help others is at major risk for burnout. Others find it easy to almost prey on this individual, and the professional can quickly become drained of personal resources. Some people will take as much as they can get and still want more. The more the professional gives to some people, the more is expected. Providers must guard against giving to excess, so that they can maintain resources for functioning on a daily basis. For many patients or clients, the best way to help is not to do everything for them, but to teach or direct them to a situation where they can acquire the skills to help themselves. Care should not be sacrificed where quality is concerned.

Individuals at high risk for burnout are often those providers who exhibit the characteristics shown in Table 12-2.

Many of these qualities are positive for the helping professions and, while people differ, it is usually those who are the most effective in the field who are most at risk for burnout, not those who are lazy or ineffectual.

Physical Signs and Symptoms of Burnout

Burnout, just like any other health problem, manifests itself in a variety of physical, emotional, and/or behavioral symptoms. In an effort to deal with potential burnout, the indicators must be recognized. Physical indicators are presented in Table 12-3.

Table 12-2   Characteristics of Individuals at High Risk for Burnout

- Motivated
- Enthusiastic/high energy
- Compassionate/sensitive
- Dedicated
- High in expectations
- Self sufficient/independent
- Impatient/have a low frustration level

Table 12-3   Physical Indicators

- Extreme fatigue or exhaustion not remedied by adequate sleep.
- Insomnia, frequent waking during the night, or the inability to fall asleep.
- Inability to go below a level 2 in the individual sleep pattern, indicating lack of deep and restful sleep.
- Frequent minor illnesses that hang on.
- Lowered resistance to infections.
- Frequent tension or migraine headaches.
- Increased blood pressure.
- Muscle tension, aches.
- Gastrointestinal disorders and loss of appetite, nausea, heartburn, ulcers.
- Generally feeling "run down" or "operating on remote."

Individuals may exhibit other physical signs of burnout specific to them. Question any that regularly appear.

Emotional Signs and Symptoms of Burnout

Emotional aspects of burnout can be as varied as the people who experience them. While the most common symptom is depression in various degrees, from mild to extreme, other signs and symptoms include those in Table 12-4.

Behavioral Signs and Symptoms of Burnout

In addition to physical and emotional indicators of burnout, behavior changes can also occur. Some of these changes may come on gradually, and for some individuals, the changes may occur over a short period of time, show up as drastic deviations from normal behavior, and draw notice from others. Behavioral signs and symptoms can include those shown in Table 12-5.

An important aspect of burnout is the tendency to rationalize. We can always come up with what seems to the individual a justification for any behavior. The bottom line, however, is that burnout poses a health risk to the professional and those individuals in the professional's care.

Stages of Burnout   Burnout typically progresses through five stages.

1. Enthusiasm. Most professionals, at least initially, are idealistic and frequently feel that they can "save the world." Enthusiasm is high and extra hours are common; the professional may tend to empathize with

---

Table 12-4   Emotional Signs and Symptoms of Burnout

- Self-doubt about job performance, professional skills, and ability to get along with people.
- Feelings of helplessness, hopelessness, or anxiety.
- Apathy/stagnation.
- A pessimistic attitude.
- Increased resistance to change, or rigidity.
- Increased hostility, frustration, resentfulness, or shortness of temper.
- Inability to concentrate/forgetfulness.
- Decreased ability to reason.
- Decreased ability to think or act quickly in an emergency.
- Increased tendency toward emotional outbursts, crying.
- Carelessness, tendency toward accident prone behaviors.
- Feelings of indispensability.

Table 12-5   Behavioral Signs and Symptoms of Burnout

- Drug use, especially tranquilizers and/or alcohol.
- Eating disorders—over-consumption of food, anorexia (self starvation), or bulimia (binge-purge).
- Negative changes in personal relationships.
- Spending longer hours at work, accomplishing less.
- Regularly sacrificing personal time to put in extra hours.
- Increased conflict at home and/or at work.
- Failure to eat lunch or take scheduled breaks or days off.
- Fault-finding with other staff members.
- Inability to compliment or enjoy others' success.
- Tendency to make multiple minor errors, and/or inappropriate defensiveness when those errors are brought up.
- Limited vision—concentrating on textbook solutions rather than using creative problem-solving.
- Frequently calling in sick, being late, leaving work early.
- Limiting time spent with patients/clients.
- Abruptness with patients/co-workers.
- Tendency to label or dehumanize patients/clients.

---

patients a great deal, mulling over patient problems in off-hours, attempting to develop suggestions that might help.

2. Stagnation. While the health care professional may still enjoy the job, enthusiasm, idealism, and motivation start to lag. The job is not what it once was; minor annoyances and aggravations start to show up that went previously unnoticed.

3. Frustration. When the individual reaches the frustration level, the two most notable occurrences are

   a) After providing for everyone else's needs for so long, the professional finally realizes that personal needs have gone unmet, perhaps for a significant period of time. The applicable influencing factors hit home, and the provider may place the blame for burnout on the patients.

   b) Physical, emotional, and behavioral signs and symptoms start to show up.

At this point, the level of frustration determines how burnout is handled. Frustration generates energy, and how that energy is used determines whether the professional goes further into the burnout process, or takes personal responsibility and control of the situation in an effort to manage burnout productively.

4. Apathy. Prolonged, unresolved frustration usually progresses to apathy. The caring professional is now only interested in personal survival, which may translate into financial survival. This stage often exaggerates the detachment that may be necessary for functioning at any level. Patients become simply a means to an end, and the provider may become very impersonal in relating to others.

5. Hopelessness. The final stage of burnout is hopelessness. Individuals typically feel that they no longer have control over their situation and, at this point, may leave their chosen profession, either temporarily or permanently. Leaving the situation does not necessarily mean that the signs and symptoms will all be resolved. Whether individuals take a leave of absence or leave the profession, individual control needs to be regained in order to ensure that personal physical and emotional health is regained.

Breaking the Cycle

Burnout is contagious, no matter what the stage. Health care providers interact closely with others on a daily basis, and attitudes and ideas have an impact. It is important to break the cycle of burnout contagion in a health care facility.

Depending upon the individual's personal qualities and the specifics of the situation, a variety of techniques can be used.

- Develop an altruistic ego. Recognize that part of the health care provider's job behind the scenes is to meet personal needs. It is necessary to be selfish sometimes, as long as it is not reckless selfishness. Keep in mind that no one can provide quality care unless they are physically and emotionally equal to the challenge. That means meeting personal needs.

- Establish some variety in the job, if possible. It will keep boredom at bay, and may offer the opportunity for professional development training. If stagnation is a problem, take a class; increase skill level in an area that is of personal or professional interest.

- Maintain a healthy diet and exercise level. Diet helps maintain nutritional health, while exercise helps work off frustration.

- Develop outside interests unrelated to the job. Health care providers who work with people all day may choose to develop their creative side using artistic mediums such as crafts, stained glass construction, painting, sewing, woodworking, writing poetry or short stories, and so on.

- Learn to say no. Individuals typically know their own needs and schedules better than anyone else. If a request is made for the provider to work extra hours, and it cannot be worked into the personal schedule, **tactfully** say so.

- Develop assertiveness skills. Be aware that this does not mean being overly aggressive.

- Learn to appreciate others and to find the positive. Each co-worker, friend, patient, or individual can give us a reason to show appreciation.

- Get away from work periodically and enjoy simple pleasures—a hot cup of coffee, stepping outside into the sunshine—and do not feel guilty about it. A regular diet of little pleasures helps maintain a positive attitude.

- Delegate where appropriate. It is usually unnecessary for one person to be responsible for absolutely everything, and no one is indispensable.

- Take a close look at what is causing stress on the job. Mark Twain once said, "I am an old man and have known a great many troubles, but most of them never happened." Most people expect problems and spend a great deal of time in worried anticipation. Murphy's Law is wrong much of the time.

- Rest. When you are tired, you are more easily stressed and less prepared to deal with productive resolution.

- Try and get away for lunch. A change of environment, preferably unhurried change, works wonders in reducing stress levels for most people.

- Maintain your personal health. Practice what you are probably preaching.

- If there is a problem, tactfully take it to the source for resolution. Nothing gets changed or dealt with if others involved do not know there may be a problem.

- When you have time off, truly make it your time. Separate work from family/personal life where possible.

- Evaluate your professional goals to make sure that they are realistic. If no goals have been established, this is the time to develop them. It is difficult to know what road to travel if you do not know the destination.

- Seek a support group or professional help if you think that it would be beneficial. An impartial sounding-board can be very helpful in discovering the particular sources of stress. It can lead to self-discovery and workable stress reduction techniques by providing a support system unavailable on the job.

If nothing seems to work after all efforts have been tried, it might be wise to seek another position in the same field, choose a related field in which to use your skills, or seek another profession. The choice is as individual as the person making it.

Summary

Stress and burnout are common problems in the helping professions, and health care providers are particularly vulnerable because of the drain on personal, physical, and emotional resources. Dealing with stress is an ongoing struggle, and burnout can occur more than once. It is important to recognize the signs and symptoms of stress and burnout so that they can be dealt with before the health professional's personal well-being and professional effectiveness are affected in a negative way.

Review Questions

1. What is the difference between distress and eustress? Give examples of each.
2. Identify and explain the four major causes of stress. How do they relate to individual daily life? Give some examples of how each type of stress affects individuals differently.
3. Explain how people react physically to stress. Are everyone's reactions the same?
4. Define the fight-or-flight response, and explain the different physical changes that occur.
5. How do epinephrine and norepinephrine affect the body during stress?
6. Why might an individual's response to stress lower the effectiveness of the immune system and leave the individual susceptible to disease?
7. What is the difference between essential hypertension and secondary hypertension?
8. What is the difference between stress and burnout?
9. Explain the productive techniques used to deal with stress.
10. Explain the nonproductive techniques used to deal with stress. As non-productive techniques, can these choices cause additional problems or stress? How?
11. Describe the characteristics of those individuals most at risk for burnout.
12. What are the physical signs and symptoms of burnout?

13. Differentiate between the emotional and the behavioral signs of burnout.
14. Describe the stages of burnout.
15. How can burnout be averted or the cycle be broken?

CHAPTER 13

Special Legal Issues

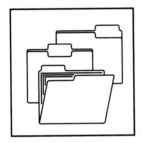

Objectives

After completing this chapter the learner should be able to:

1. Define the Good Samaritan law.
2. Define standard of care.
3. List situations where the Good Samaritan law does not apply.
4. Define **respondeat superior.**
5. Describe how an office emergency can be dangerous to personnel.
6. List general guidelines to avoid the dangers of rendering emergency care beyond scope of training limits.
7. Define medical malpractice.
8. Describe the importance of purchasing liability insurance.
9. List four areas of importance in considering purchasing a malpractice policy.
10. Define living will and life-prolonging declarations.
11. List general laws for living wills.
12. List ethical and legal issues surrounding the living will.
13. Define organ and tissue donation.

14. Describe who is eligible for organ and tissue donation.
15. Describe how organs are obtained.

Introduction

This chapter includes legal issues that the health care professional will have to deal with in the medical office. Each member should be aware of potential legal problems and be knowledgeable in providing information to patients if they request it. The application of the Good Samaritan law as it applies to the medical office, professional liability, living wills, and tissue and organ donations is also discussed in this chapter.

Good Samaritan Laws

Good Samaritan laws were created to protect the health care professional who, off-duty, might stop and render first aid in an emergency situation. While all 50 states have a Good Samaritan law, it should be noted that the content varies widely in each of the individual states. In Indiana the law covers any person, regardless of profession, who stops to render care, but in other states there are separate Good Samaritan laws for nurses. All medical professionals should become familiar with their state's statute.

In the majority of states, the decision to provide care in an off-duty situation is voluntary. The Good Samaritan law is intended to protect those professionals who stop to render first-aid care in good faith and without gross negligence. Health care professionals would not be legally liable if they chose not to stop and render care. However, if the decision to stop is made, the health care professional incurs a legal duty. The professional is legally responsible for the victim and may not leave unless the victim is being cared for by another health care professional with at least as much training, or until police order the rescuer from the scene. It is important to realize that from the moment of stopping, a duty to provide assistance is established based on the standard of care of a reasonably prudent health care professional in a similar situation.

The rescuer will be judged by his/her actions according to rescuer training and experience. The level of care provided must not exceed the scope of training and not fall below the usual standard of care given. Treatment given that exceeds the individual's training may cause that individual to be judged to a higher standard of care. That is to say, a medical assistant who performs like a paramedic can be judged according to what a paramedic is expected to know.

Remember that Good Samaritan laws act to limit the liability that can be associated with stopping at the scene of an accident. There have been few health care professionals sued as a result of providing care. The Good Samaritan laws do not apply to individuals who are providing emergency care while on the job. The laws were designed to help protect health care professionals when providing off-duty emergency care. The safest way to avoid liability is to always stay within your scope of training.

Many of the Good Samaritan laws are poorly written and do not have definite meanings for the terms included in the document. Questions that are left unanswered include:

- What is meant by "graciously"?
- What is the definition of an emergency?
- When does the care given exceed the law?

In addition, the ethical issues of rendering emergency care need to be addressed. The American Medical Association advises physicians to respond to any requests for assistance in an emergency. The legal and ethical issues should be considered before an emergency situation arises.

Professional Liability

The doctrine of **respondeat superior** is a Latin phrase that means, "Let the master answer." Legally, physicians are professionally liable for not only their own actions, but also the negligent actions of their employees when they are officially on the job. The medical office personnel must be careful to function within the scope of their knowledge and training. Negligent acts of employees can result in both civil and criminal charges being brought against the physician employer.

General Guidelines for Scope of Training Limits

An emergency situation is an especially dangerous time for office personnel. In their need to assist the patient, they may be tempted to go beyond the scope of their training. To avoid this pitfall, these general guidelines should be followed before dealing with emergency situations:

1. The medical office personnel and the physician need to have clearly established protocols for dealing with emergencies.
    Rationale: If the office personnel know what their role is, they are less likely to deviate from it.

2. Each person in the office should receive training in CPR and basic first aid.
   Rationale: Individuals who, through formal training, feel confident in providing cardiopulmonary resuscitation are less likely to go beyond the training received.

3. All individuals in the office should know their own state's restrictions on practicing in their profession.
   Rationale: Each state has its own laws dealing with different professionals.

Following these guidelines may help the medical personnel to avoid allegations of malpractice.

Medical malpractice is defined as doing or not doing something a reasonable and prudent person would or would not do. In cases of emergencies, it is often difficult to have the necessary time to evaluate the situation. However, it is possible to have a properly trained team that can respond to emergencies efficiently and effectively.

Malpractice Insurance

Because every situation in a medical office could result in a lawsuit, every member should purchase liability insurance. **Respondeat superior** and the malpractice insurance the physician carries are not sufficient protection, given the legal risks associated with providing today's health care. In order to be assured that the physician has purchased adequate insurance, the employee should be familiar with the physician's policy. Areas of the policy to review are:

1. Coverage limits. What is maximum dollar coverage?
2. Threshold limit. This term refers to a dollar amount (usually $3,000) that allows the insurer to settle a case without the employee's permission. If the amount is above the threshold limit, the insurer must have the employee's permission. Settling out of court could jeopardize your professional reputation.
3. Stipulations for denying coverage. The policy may contain a time limit or exclusion.
4. Claims policy. This policy only covers employees if they are still employed at the time of the claim.

The purchase of malpractice insurance should be discussed with an agent familiar with this type of insurance coverage. Usually the agent will review the employer policy without charge in order to provide the employee with the most comprehensive coverage. Cost will vary with the type of policy purchased, but it can usually be purchased for less than $100 a year—a relatively small cost compared to losing all personal property if sued successfully.

Living Wills

With today's advanced technology, everyone should be aware of the need for a living will. Medical technology can keep people alive well beyond what was once possible. Indeed, this ability poses many ethical and legal problems for today's society as a whole. The living will is a document that informs doctors, family members, hospitals, and, most importantly, the courts what a patient's wishes are if the patient becomes unable to direct the extent of care (see Fig 13-1). There is also a document, called the Life-Prolonging Procedures Declaration, that instructs the physician to do everything possible to maintain life.

General Guidelines for Living Will

Each state has unique statutory requirements, so medical office personnel should become familiar with their state's laws. The laws will generally:

1. Indicate the persons authorized to make a living will (usually restricted to a competent adult).
2. Define the circumstances under which a living will can apply.
3. Define limitations of the will concerning care that can be refused.
4. Define witnessing requirements.
5. List procedures for rescinding a living will.
6. Identify liability immunity for following a living will's directives.

The office should be sure that, if a patient has a living will, a copy is kept in the patient's file. Both the living will and the life-prolonging declaration are methods that allow adults to control their medical treatment decisions even if incapacitated. Decisions to provide, withhold, or withdraw treatment often have to be made late in an illness or injury. It is a document that states the patient's desires for what type of medical care is to be received. The use of surgeries, radiation, artificial respirators, and forced feeding can be avoided by the use of a living will.

The life-prolonging declaration is the opposite of the living will. It directs the physician to use any or all life-prolonging procedures, no matter how extraordinary the cost or care. The patient must be competent and two witnesses

THE FOLLOWING IS AN EXAMPLE OF A LIVING WILL FOR THE STATE OF FLORIDA. PLEASE CONTACT CHOICE IN DYING AT (800) 989-WILL TO RECEIVE A FREE COPY OF APPROPRIATE ADVANCE DIRECTIVES FOR YOUR STATE.

FLORIDA LIVING WILL

INSTRUCTIONS

PRINT THE DATE

Declaration made this _____ day of _____, 19_____.

PRINT YOUR NAME

I, _____, willfully and voluntarily make known my desire that my dying not be artificially prolonged under the circumstances set forth below, and I do hereby declare:

If at any time I have a terminal condition and if my attending or treating physician and another consulting physician have determined that there is no medical probability of my recovery from such condition, I direct that life-prolonging procedures be withheld or withdrawn when the application of such procedures would serve only to prolong artificially the process of dying, and that I be permitted to die naturally with only the administration of medication or the performance of any medical procedure deemed necessary to provide me with comfort care or to alleviate pain.

It is my intention that this declaration be honored by my family and physician as the final expression of my legal right to refuse medical or surgical treatment and to accept the consequences for such refusal.

In the event that I have been determined to be unable to provide express and informed consent regarding the withholding, withdrawal, or continuation of life-prolonging procedures, I wish to designate, as my surrogate to carry out the provisions of this declaration:

PRINT THE NAME, HOME ADDRESS AND TELEPHONE NUMBER OF YOUR SURROGATE

Name: _____

Address: _____

_____ Zip Code: _____

Phone: _____

© 1993
CHOICE IN DYING, INC.

Figure 13-1a Living will declaration. Choice In Dying makes available legally recognized document forms to residents of states that have enacted right-to-die laws. For people in states that have not enacted right-to-die laws, Choice In Dying provides statutory advance directives for each state free of charge, as well as other materials and services relating to end-of-life medical care. (Reprinted by permission of Choice In Dying, 200 Varick Street, New York, New York 10014, 212-366-5540.)

I wish to designate the following person as my alternate surrogate, to carry out the provisions of this declaration should my surrogate be unwilling or unable to act on my behalf:

PRINT NAME, HOME ADDRESS AND TELEPHONE NUMBER OF YOUR ALTERNATE SURROGATE

Name: _____

Address: _____

_____ Zip Code: _____

Phone: _____

ADD PERSONAL INSTRUCTIONS (IF ANY)

Additional instructions (optional):

I understand the full import of this declaration, and I am emotionally and mentally competent to make this declaration.

SIGN THE DOCUMENT

Signed: _____

WITNESSING PROCEDURE

Witness 1:

TWO WITNESSES MUST SIGN AND PRINT THEIR ADDRESSES

   Signed: _____

   Address: _____

Witness 2:

   Signed: _____

   Address: _____

© 1993
CHOICE IN DYING, INC.

Courtesy of Choice In Dying   11/93
200 Varick Street, New York, NY 10014 1-800-989-WILL

PAGE 2

Figure 13-1b   *Continued.*

must be present during the signing of the will. Witnesses need not be parents, spouses, children, or anyone who will benefit from the patient's estate.

Several states have a Health Care Consent Act that allows the patient to appoint someone to make their health care decisions if the patient becomes incapable of doing so (see Figure 13-2). An attorney needs to prepare the form to be sure that the correct language is used, or contact Choice In Dying, Inc. to receive appropriate advance directives for your state. The representative cannot overrule a patient's previous instruction, such as a living will.

Every state has different versions of the Health Care Surrogate form and the requirements for filling them out. Health care professionals should become familiar with what is standard in their state.

While the living will is not a legal document, it does clarify and communicate the patient's wishes, an important element in ethical issues of patient care. Patients should be encouraged to verbalize their wishes with family and friends. An understanding and acceptance by the individual's family will help to ensure their compliance with the patient's wishes.

Organ and Tissue Donation

During the past 30 years, organ and tissue transplants have become possible. Surgeons are able to transplant successfully about 25 different organs and tissues, which include cornea, kidney, heart, lung, pancreas, liver, bone marrow, and skin. Improved surgical techniques, new drugs to help fight rejection, and better postoperative care are providing a better success rate for these transplants.

Required Request or Routine Inquiry

There is a serious shortage of organs to provide patients with a new chance of life. In 1987 the federal government passed a "required request or routine inquiry" by all hospitals to help increase the availability of organs and tissues. The purpose of this legislation is to require hospitals to develop a system to identify potential organ and tissue donors at the time of death. The law requires the physician or hospital staff member to ask whether or not the family of the identified patient has considered organ and tissue donation. Whether or not a donation is made is up to the family.

To understand the magnitude of the shortage of organs and tissues, there are at any time at least 8,500 people waiting for kidneys, 250 for livers, 100 for hearts, and at least 4,000 for corneas.

THE FOLLOWING IS AN EXAMPLE OF A FORM USED TO DESIGNATE A
HEALTH CARE AGENT IN THE STATE OF FLORIDA. PLEASE CONTACT
CHOICE IN DYING AT (800) 989-WILL TO RECEIVE A FREE COPY
OF APPROPRIATE ADVANCE DIRECTIVES FOR YOUR STATE.

INSTRUCTIONS

FLORIDA DESIGNATION OF HEALTH CARE SURROGATE

PRINT YOUR NAME

Name: _____
   (Last)   (First)   (Middle Initial)

In the event that I have been determined to be incapacitated to provide informed consent for medical treatment and surgical and diagnostic procedures, I wish to designate as my surrogate for health care decisions:

PRINT THE NAME, HOME ADDRESS AND TELEPHONE NUMBER OF YOUR SURROGATE

Name: _____

Address: _____

_____ Zip Code: _____

Phone: _____

If my surrogate is unwilling or unable to perform his duties, I wish to designate as my alternate surrogate:

PRINT THE NAME, HOME ADDRESS AND TELEPHONE NUMBER OF YOUR ALTERNATE SURROGATE

Name: _____

Address: _____

_____ Zip Code: _____

Phone: _____

I fully understand that this designation will permit my designee to make health care decisions and to provide, withhold, or withdraw consent on my behalf; to apply for public benefits to defray the cost of health care; and to authorize my admission to or transfer from a health care facility.

© 1993
CHOICE IN DYING, INC.

Figure 13-2a Health Care Surrogate Form. (Reprinted by permission of Choice In Dying, 200 Varick Street, New York, New York 10014, 212-366-5540.)

ADD PERSONAL INSTRUCTIONS (IF ANY)	Additional instructions (optional):

I further affirm that this designation is not being made as a condition of treatment or admission to a health care facility. I will notify and send a copy of this document to the following persons other than my surrogate, so they may know who my surrogate is:

PRINT THE NAMES AND ADDRESSES OF THOSE WHO YOU WANT TO KEEP COPIES OF THIS DOCUMENT

Name: _____

Address: _____

Name: _____

Address: _____

SIGN AND DATE THE DOCUMENT

Signed: _____

Date: _____

WITNESSING PROCEDURE

TWO WITNESSES MUST SIGN AND PRINT THEIR ADDRESSES

Witness 1:

   Signed: _____

   Address: _____

Witness 2:

   Signed: _____

   Address: _____

SAMPLE

© 1993
CHOICE IN DYING, INC.

Courtesy of Choice In Dying   11/93
200 Varick Street, New York, NY 10014 1-800-989-WILL

PAGE 2

Figure 13-2a   *Continued.*

General Guidelines for Donations

General information concerning organ or tissue donations are:

1. Eligibility criteria are different for each case. The ideal donor is a healthy individual who has suffered irreversible central nervous system injury. Accidents most commonly associated with this type of injury are motorcycle and auto accidents, gunshot wounds, stabbings, drug overdose, electrocution, suffocation, and drowning.

2. In most cases, it is a federal offense to sell organs in the United States. Hospitals, donors, or donors' heirs may not receive payment for organs or tissues.

3. In most cases, there is no charge for donating or procuring the organs and tissues. Families of organ or tissue donors are not charged.

4. Many private insurance companies cover the cost of transplants. In 1986 Medicare began to cover the cost of heart and liver transplants. Medicare will also cover liver transplants in individuals under the age of 18 who have biliary atresia or rare, selected liver diseases.

5. Medicaid, which is administered on a state basis, covers transplants for heart, heart/lung, liver, and kidney. Only four states pay for pancreas transplants.

6. There is a 24-hour national computer-alert system that provides information on patients waiting for organ donations, allowing for quick matches of donor and recipients.

7. Additional information about organ and tissue donation can be obtained from:
   The American Council on Transplantation
   4701 Willard Avenue
   Suite 222
   Chevy Chase, Maryland 20815
   (301) 652-0094

Summary

Health care professionals need to remember that the Good Samaritan laws are no guarantee that they will not be sued. Good Samaritan laws vary in each state and may not apply in all situations. The best protection for health care professionals is to be familiar with their own state laws.

Unfortunately, malpractice suits are more frequent today than in the past. Certainly dealing with emergencies in the office increases the risk. A well-prepared team that knows the laws of the state can reduce those risks. Because of these risks, every team member should consider purchasing malpractice insurance for peace of mind and financial protection.

Living wills, life-prolonging documents, and organ and tissue donations are very delicate issues that should be addressed by the health care staff. Patients need to be informed of how and why these decisions and documents must be completed before a serious illness or injury develops. At the very least, it is the responsibility of the medical office to be aware of these documents and their uses.

Review Questions

1. What emergencies need to be considered in advance of an emergency situation?
2. How does an emergency in the office differ from one "on the street"?
3. Explain the Good Samaritan law.
4. When is the doctrine of **respondeat superior** used? Give an example.
5. List the guidelines for avoiding liability.
6. Why is going beyond an individual's scope of training dangerous?
7. Define medical malpractice.
8. Explain coverage limits and threshold limits.
9. Do you or any members of your family have a living will? If so, why or why not?
10. Discuss with others your feelings concerning this issue.
11. List at least 2 legal and/or ethical issues regarding this topic.
12. List organs and tissues that can be transplanted.
13. Describe the "ideal donor."
14. Explain who pays the cost of transplantation.

CHAPTER 14

Legal Documentation

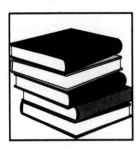

Objectives

After completing this chapter the learner should be able to:

1. Describe why maintaining a patient's chart is necessary.
2. List 6 questions that medical personnel should ask themselves.
3. Define the "rule of thumb" when charting.
4. Describe the impact documentation has on a malpractice suit.
5. List 4 situations that require special documentation.
6. Describe what a refusal-of-treatment form is and when it is used.
7. Describe what should be done when a living will is brought to the office.
8. List 6 guidelines used when dealing with verbal orders.
9. List what elements should be included when documenting an emergency situation.

Introduction

The patient chart is the road map of the treatment received by the patient. It tells why the patient has come to the office, diagnosis, the care given, and any plans made for future care and testing. This chart is considered a legal document and can provide information for malpractice, work-related disability claims, Medicare auditing, and personal injury lawsuits.

The chart must reflect a complete and accurate description of all services provided to the patient by the office. This chart can be subpoenaed by the courts in cases of malpractice or other litigation cases, and it can provide legal protection to the office.

Documentation is required to provide a written description of the patient's care by the medical office. Medicare, for example, requires that offices provide evidence (in the form of documentation) that the treatment is directly related to the diagnosis. Failure to provide adequate documentation can result in a fine, and possible loss of Medicare privileges. States require documentation of births, deaths, and certain infectious diseases.

General Guidelines

When adding information to a patient's chart, be sure to keep the following in mind:

1. Does the charting accurately reflect what happened?
2. Is the charting in chronological order?
3. Is there adequate description to cover events?
4. Has the appropriate terminology been used?
5. Is the charting neat and easy to read?
6. If there were errors made, are they corrected properly?

Improper charting can confuse a reader at a later date. When charting, chart each entry as if a third party will be reading the chart at some time.

Sometimes the office personnel may be in doubt as to what information to record and what to leave out. A good rule of thumb is, when in doubt, chart everything. Failing to record information can result in misunderstandings and can jeopardize the quality of a patient's care.

In malpractice suits, the patient's attorney will attempt to prove that a standard of care was not met. Documentation that is incomplete or illegible makes the opposing attorney's job that much easier. Often the absence of any documentation can prove the patient's allegations.

Special Documentation

Certain situations, including verifying patient consent, patient refusal of treatment, handling legal wills, and taking verbal orders, will require special treatment.

Consent

When dealing with an emergency situation, personnel should always ask permission of the conscious patient or family, if present. The office personnel should use a standard dialogue that is documented in an office procedures manual and again in the individual patient chart. Here is an example: "I know what to do; can I help you?" Then proceed to explain to the patient just exactly what you will be doing. This consent can be waived when the patient is unconscious or when the patient is a minor and you have the guardian's consent to proceed.

In addition, the patient has the right to refuse treatment. The legal system today recognizes that a competent adult has the right to refuse treatment, even if that refusal will result in death. Documentation should include the patient's exact words and that the patient was fully informed about the medical condition and the likely consequences of the refusal. Ask the patient to sign a refusal-of-treatment release form. If the patient refuses to sign, document the refusal (see Figure 14-1).

Living Will

The office should include specific information on the development of living wills in the office procedure manual. Carefully document the circumstances surrounding the living will and how the situation was handled. A flag should be put on the outside of the patient's chart when it contains a living will document.

Verbal Orders

When dealing in an emergency situation, verbal orders are a necessity. Documenting verbal orders can be a liability problem for the office. Every precaution must be taken to insure the accuracy of the documentation in this situation. General guidelines are:

1. Assign one member of the staff to document during the emergency.
2. All verbal orders should be repeated immediately back to the doctor.
3. If no one is present to document during the emergency, record the orders as soon as possible after the emergency.
4. Be sure to write "V.O." for verbal order and have the doctor initial the orders.

REFUSAL-OF-TREATMENT RELEASE FORM

I _____ refuse to allow Dr.
                        Patient's name

_____ and staff to administer
                        Doctor's name

_____ to me.
                        Treatment

The risks involved in refusing treatment have been explained to me and I fully understand the consequences of my actions.

I hereby release the doctor and the doctor's staff from liability for respecting and following my express wishes and directions.

_____   _____
Witness signature   Patient's or legal guardian's
                                              signature

_____   _____
Date   Patient's age

Figure 14-1 Refusal-of-Treatment Release Form

5. Be sure to sign the record, write the time the emergency occurred, and note what time the documentation was done.

6. Draw lines through any spaces between the order and the verification of the order.

Documenting information concerning the patient and incidences that occurred in the office can be essential in proving what type of care was given. Often the medical record is seen as the most credible evidence available; it can be either the best defense for the office or can substantiate the patient's charges. Poor documentation can make a competently handled emergency appear incomplete and negligent.

Documentation of an emergency should include all medical treatment given, patient's comments, personal appearance, vital signs (including how often they were taken), medications administered (strength, dosage, rate, and route), if and how much oxygen was administered, and who was present during the emergency. Include any family comments. Remember: When in doubt about whether or not to chart it, chart it.

Summary

An accurate description of what took place during an emergency situation can be the best defense to allegations of malpractice. Office personnel must protect themselves by keeping careful records on patient care.

Review Questions

1. What is the purpose of documentation?
2. What information do state governments require to be accurately documented?
3. What is the purpose of documentation in regard to malpractice suits?
4. What is the "rule of thumb" to be used when charting?
5. When might a refusal-of-treatment form be required? Is it necessary to document refusal of treatment? Why or why not?
6. What should be done when a living will is brought to the office?
7. Identify and explain the 6 guidelines that should be used when dealing with verbal orders.
8. What elements should be included when documenting an emergency?

CHAPTER 15

Recognizing Victims of Abuse or Neglect

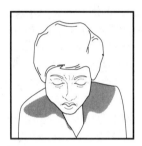

Objectives

After completing this chapter the learner should be able to:

1. Explain why health care professionals need to be aware of the signs and symptoms of abusive behavior.

2. Identify and explain the 9 most typical characteristics of adults most at risk for becoming abusive or neglectful.

3. Identify the most common life crises or stressors that can influence an individual's "trigger" for abusive or neglectful behaviors.

Introduction

Victims of abuse are an often overlooked part of our society. Unless an individual's injuries are severe enough to warrant immediate concern, health care providers often do not attempt to offer assistance to the victim or the family. Frequently, health care providers are unaware of the signs and symptoms of abuse, and lack the knowledge to identify what constitutes the professional's reporting responsibilities. Health care professionals need to learn to identify possible victims of various types of abuse and neglect. In order to facilitate the best possible care, the professional should also become familiar with techniques for handling the physical, emotional, and legal aspects of abuse and neglect.

In any given year, about half of the households in the United States are the scene of some type of family violence or abusive behavior. There is no certain way to determine **exactly** how extensive abuse and neglect are because much of it is never reported or identified. The situation(s) may involve a parent or caregiver hitting a child, a spouse striking his/her partner, violence between siblings, or a child being abusive toward a parent.

The best way to provide assistance is to understand the various factors involved, to recognize that **anyone,** under certain circumstances, can be the perpetrator of abuse, as well as a victim, and to be aware of methods and legalities for handling the situation. Abusive behaviors cross all social, economic, age, gender, racial, and ethnic boundaries. It is important that everyone understand that abuse is **never** appropriate, and no one is an appropriate victim, regardless of the circumstances. Abuse and neglect are community problems that require community solutions. Learning the signs and symptoms of abuse and neglect will enable health care providers to identify an individual at risk and to offer services and/or referrals to the individual or family before further damage can occur.

Typical Characteristics of Individuals at Risk for Becoming Abusive

Everyone has certain "triggers" or stimuli that provoke an immediate negative reaction. Based on individual differences and experiences, some caregivers or partners may be more at risk than others for becoming abusive. The most typical characteristics of individuals at risk for becoming abusive include:

Poor Childhood Experiences

Adults who were abused or neglected as children may repeat the pattern with their own children. This appears to be "normal" behavior because it may be all the adult has ever experienced. If the individual consistently witnessed physical and/or emotional violence or neglect in the family environment, this behavior may also be seen as normal, and the behaviors may be perpetuated in subsequent generations.

Immaturity

Young and/or insecure adults may have a difficult time working within a relationship at a mature level. The individual's personal needs may be significant enough that they may not be able to help meet the needs of anyone else, whether that is a child or another adult.

Unrealistic Expectations

Where children are concerned, the caregiver may be unaware of the normal stages of child development, and may expect behaviors from a child that the child is not capable of understanding or performing at that particular point of development. Children are not short adults. They lack the experience and the time, part of the adult's growth and maturation process, to develop physically, emotionally, and intellectually.

In establishing relationships with other adults, it is sometimes easy to slip into expecting too much from someone else. Everyone has different skills and abilities, and expecting someone else to conform to a personal idea of perfection is unrealistic. Life is under no obligation to give us what we expect, and when outside influences must be dealt with, it is necessary to adapt. Adaptation skills are learned skills.

Lack of Parenting Skills

In working with or raising children, parenting/caregiving skills often must be learned. If the adults did not learn to parent through exposure to good skills while they were being raised, outside training or education should be sought. Good parenting skills rarely come naturally without exposure to good examples of such skills.

Unmet Emotional Needs

Adults who do not relate well to other adults may expect children to satisfy their needs for love, protection, self-esteem, and importance. Individuals may also expect other significant adults in their life to provide these things to validate their existence and value.

Isolation

Individuals who have little or no support system may take their frustration out on the individual(s) closest to them, regardless of whether that includes children or another adult. This isolation can be geographical or emotional.

Substance Abuse

According to the Office for Substance Abuse Prevention (OSAP), alcohol and other drugs are associated with 38 percent of reported cases of child abuse, up to 50 percent of spouse abuse cases, 52 percent of rapes, and 62 percent of assault incidents. Substance use/abuse limits the ability of the individual to think and reason clearly and to adapt appropriately to any given situation.

Mental Illness or Developmental Delay

Individuals with an unstable psychological makeup or low intellectual functioning may not fully understand the range of responsibilities associated with parenting or with maintaining good adult relationships. This lack of understanding may show up in abusive or neglectful behaviors.

The Acceptance of Violence in Our Society

Each day our population is exposed to a number of violent acts; acts of violence are alluded to either verbally or by threating actions, and the media plays a major role in this exposure. Movies, television, magazines, and radio all portray different aspects of violence, and portray a variety of racial, ethnic, socio-economic, age, and gender groups as victims. Violence is no longer the deviation in behavior or problem solving skills. In many instances, violence is viewed as an acceptable way to handle conflict and release frustration and aggression.

Given the 9 characteristics identified as possible factors for contributing to an individual's risk of becoming abusive or neglectful, it is imperative that the professional understand that not all abusive adults exhibit these characteristics. Likewise, not everyone who has been raised in an abusive or neglectful environment perpetuates those behaviors. Be wary of making blanket judgments.

Life Crises or Stressors

Even under the best of circumstances, changes can occur that are unplanned or unanticipated. Any significant disruption in the lifestyle or individual's normal way of life can increase stress and contribute to an abusive outburst or lack of care. The most common life crises or stressors include those listed in Table 15-1.

Victims of abuse and neglect fall into a variety of age ranges, as do the perpetrators of abuse and neglect. A number of types of abuse have been identified, and the medical professional should be aware of the signs and symptoms of each one, as well as professional and legal responsibilities involved.

The next two chapters will discuss child physical, sexual, and emotional abuse, Munchausen's Syndrome and Munchausen's Syndrome by Proxy, child physical and emotional neglect, Shaken Baby Syndrome, Sudden Infant Death

Table 15-1   Common Life Crises or Stressors

- Death of a loved one.
- Divorce.
- Loss of a job/source of income.
- Major illness or injury to the individual or another significant person in their life.
- A chaotic lifestyle.
- An accumulation of small, everyday stresses, frustrations, and annoyances.

Syndrome (SIDS), Osteogenesis Imperfecta, adult physical and sexual abuse, rape, elder maltreatment, and self-neglect.

Summary

Health care professionals should be aware of the signs and symptoms of the various types of abuse and should be familiar with the characteristics of and influences on abusive or neglectful situations. Essentially, under certain circumstances, anyone can be a perpetrator of abuse or neglect, and anyone can be a victim. The professional should be familiar with community resources in order to make reports and/or referrals for assistance.

Review Questions

1. Explain why it is helpful for health care professionals to learn the signs and symptoms of abusive behavior.
2. Identify and explain the nine characteristics of individuals who are considered to be at risk for becoming abusive.
3. What life crises or stressors influence abusive or neglectful situations?

CHAPTER 16

Child Abuse and Neglect

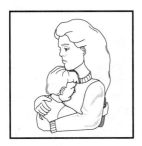

Objectives

After completing this chapter the learner should be able to:

1. Identify the characteristics of children who are typically at increased risk for being abused or neglected.

2. Identify the general effects of abuse and/or neglect on the child.

3. Explain the physical indicators of child physical abuse.

4. Explain the criteria for dating bruises.

5. Define: Shaken Baby Syndrome
             Munchausen's Syndrome by Proxy
             Osteogenesis Imperfecta
             Sudden Infant Death Syndrome (SIDS)

6. Differentiate between osteogenesis imperfecta congenital and osteogenesis imperfecta tarda.

7. Identify behavioral characteristics that may be exhibited by children who are victims of physical abuse.

8. Define physical neglect.

9. Identify behavioral characteristics of children who are being neglected.

10. Explain child sexual abuse.

11. Identify the physical indicators of child sexual abuse.

12. Identify typical behaviors of a child who is being sexually abused.

13. Differentiate between emotional abuse and emotional neglect.

14. Identify behavioral indicators of children who are victims of emotional maltreatment.

15. Explain the behaviors indicative of caregivers who are emotionally or psychologically abusive.

16. Define false reporting.

Introduction

In an April 1993 report of a 50-state survey, the National Committee for the Prevention of Child Abuse (NCPCA) estimated that 2,936,000 children (under the age of 18) were reported to child protective service or social service agencies as being abused or neglected in 1992. Of this number, approximately 1,160,400 cases of child abuse or neglect were substantiated, which means that there was enough evidence to support the reported claims. Of the substantiated reports, 27 percent involved physical abuse, 17 percent sexual abuse, 45 percent neglect, 7 percent emotional abuse, and 4 percent other types of abuse, which include abandonment and dependency. NCPCA also reports that approximately 1,261 children died of abuse or neglect in 1992, with 84 percent of the victims being under the age of 5, and 43 percent of those under the age of 1.

There is a continually developing awareness that child abuse and neglect are significant problems, and those that are the easiest to harm are the least able to help themselves. By recognizing the signs of abuse and neglect, knowing when and what questions to ask, and knowing what the health care professional's reporting responsibilities and resources are, it will be possible to help more children and their families.

Characteristics of Children at Increased Risk

Some children have specific characteristics that place them more at risk for abuse and neglect than others. Included would be those children whose care may pose particular difficulties for the parents or caregiver (see Table 16-1).

The Characteristics identified in Table 16-1 do not mean that those are the **only** children at risk. **Any** child has the potential for becoming abused or neglected. Likewise, however, not all children who exhibit these characteristics are being abused or neglected. Many have loving and nurturing environments in which to grow and develop.

Table 16-1   Characteristics of Children at Increased Risk of Abuse

- Children who are physically or mentally handicapped.
- Infants who have been born prematurely.
- Children who are demanding or whiny.
- Children who are hyperactive or have attention deficit disorder (ADD).
- Infants with feeding difficulties.
- Infants who are colicky or children who are illness prone.
- Children who are exceptionally bright.
- Children who are "perceived" as difficult.
- Children who may not be of the gender that the parents had hoped for.
- Children who are seen as bad, ugly, stupid, or stubborn, even if their appearance and behavior appear normal to others.
- Children who have physical or personality characteristics similar to those of someone who has caused distress to the caregiver.
- Children whose conception or birth caused particular problems.

General Effects of Abuse or Neglect

Child abuse and neglect can result in serious and permanent damage to the child. When we consider the long-term effects of abuse and neglect, the physical effects are usually the first to come to mind because the physical damage can be seen.

Physical Effects of Abuse and/or Neglect

Physical abuse can cause damage to the brain, eyes, other senses, vital internal organs, or limbs and may result in permanent disability for the child. Physical neglect can put the child at risk because of prolonged exposure to heat or cold; lack of physical care can contribute to physical illness; inadequate supervision frequently leads to accidental injuries; lack of stimulation often results in the child's failure to thrive. Physical abuse and neglect can lead to the death of the child.

Emotional Effects of Abuse and/or Neglect

All forms of abuse or neglect have a negative effect on the child's emotional health. The extent of damage depends on the type of abuse or neglect, the duration of time involved, the developmental stage of the child, the presence or absence of positive influences in the child's life, and individual differences among children. The emotional effects of abuse or neglect include low self-esteem or lack of self-esteem, poor self-image, poor social skills, difficulty in trusting others, problems in forming positive relationships, and difficulty with reality testing and thought processes.

Developmental Effects of Abuse and/or Neglect

Another effect of abuse or neglect shows itself in the form of developmental lags. As well as the possible physical damage, stimulation deprivation does nothing to encourage normal development. The child may channel significant energy into avoiding abuse. These circumstances decrease the opportunity and ability of the child to develop normally.

Physical Abuse

Physical abuse of children involves any non-accidental physical injury caused by the child's caregiver. That caregiver could be the child's parent(s), babysitter, another professional, or any responsible individual who has been entrusted with

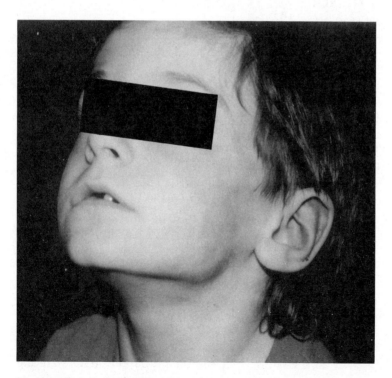

Figure 16-1   A 5-year-old child with bruises from being kicked in the face and ear.

the care of the child. Physical abuse can be the result of an intentional action meant to harm the child, or it can be the result of overzealous or inappropriate discipline.

Physical Indicators

Indicators of physical abuse may show up as **unexplained or unusual** bruises or welts, particularly:

- On the face, lips, or mouth (see Figure 16-1).
- On the torso, back, buttocks, or thighs (see Figure 16-2).
- In various stages of healing.
- Clustered, forming regular patterns.
- Reflecting the shape of the article used to cause the injury, such as a belt or belt buckle, electrical cord, or paddle.

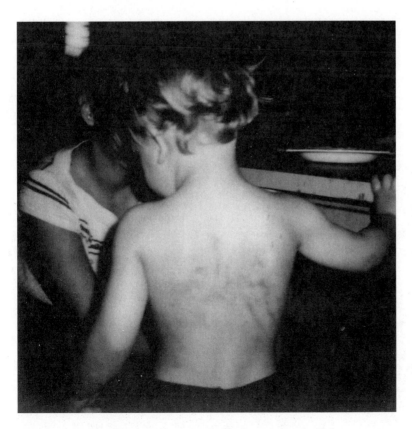

Figure 16-2   This 3-year-old was beaten with a wet wash cloth.

- On several different surface areas.
- Regularly appearing after absences, weekends, or vacations.

Dating Bruises   It is possible to approximate the age of a bruise by checking the condition and color of the bruise (see Table 16-2). Most bruises take from 2–4 weeks to disappear completely.

Unexplained Burns   The following types of burns may be suspicious if unexplained:

- Immersion burns, resembling socks or gloves, or donut-shaped burns on the buttocks or genitals (see Figure 16-3).
- Cigar or cigarette burns, especially on the soles of the feet, on the palms of the hands, between the fingers, on the back, or on the buttocks.

Table 16-2   Dating Bruises

Less than 2 days old	Area is swollen, tender, and red in color.
1–3 days old	Red, blue, or dark purple in color.
4–7 days old	Green in color.
7–14 days old	Yellow in color.
More than 2 weeks old	Brown in color.

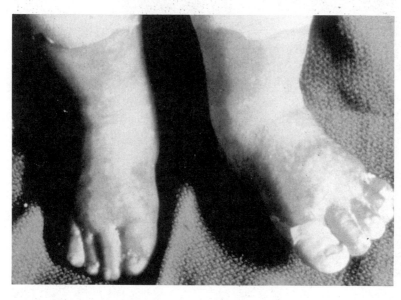

Figure 16-3   Immersion burn.

■ Burns that reflect the shape of the object causing the burn (see Figure 16-4).

Unexplained Fractures The following conditions or fractures may be suspicious if unexplained:

■ In various stages of healing.

■ To the skull, nose, or facial structure.

■ Multiple long bone fractures.

■ Spiral fractures (caused by twisting).

■ Injuries to the growth centers of the bones.

Unexplained Lacerations or Abrasions The following lacerations or abrasions may be suspicious if unexplained:

■ To the mouth, lips, gums, soft palate, eyes.

■ To external genitalia.

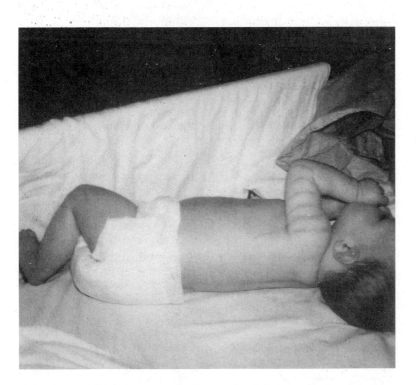

Figure 16-4 This infant was left alone and rolled onto a hot heating grate, acquiring burns on the arm and leg.

- ■ To the limbs, back, chest, or abdomen.
- ■ Ruptured frenulum (fold of mucous membrane extending from the middle of the inner surface of the lip to the area near the gums, seen in both upper and lower jaws).

Shaken Baby Syndrome

Shaken baby syndrome is seen in abused infants and children. The child has been shaken violently, with whiplash type motions; the injuries that result from the shaking can be fatal.

Medical literature started discussing shaken baby syndrome in the early 1970s. It may be part of a pattern of abuse, or it may happen because an adult succumbs to the momentary frustration of dealing with a crying infant. For a long time, doctors failed to recognize shaken baby syndrome as a cause of bleeding in the brain because there were no external signs of injury. Doctors saw only the results, most frequently brain damage, convulsions, and sometimes death.

Violent shaking of infants and young children is especially dangerous because neck muscles are undeveloped, and the brain is fragile. Vigorous shaking repeatedly jars the brain in several directions, increasing the possibility of damage. This sudden shaking motion can cause some parts of the brain to tear loose from the surrounding support work, and brain cells can be damaged in the process.

The injuries that typically result from shaking a baby or young child too hard include those shown in Table 16-3.

Shaken baby syndrome is a form of child abuse and should be recognized as such.

Munchausen's Syndrome by Proxy

In recent years a form of child abuse has been identified that is different from what has typically been defined as abuse. In Munchausen's Syndrome by Proxy, an adult caregiver takes actions to cause a child to be ill, resulting in extensive medical care for the child, including hospitalization and surgery. Examples

---

Table 16-3   Shaken Baby Syndrome Injuries

- Brain swelling and brain damage.
- Subdural hemorrhage.
- Mental retardation.
- Blindness, or vision impairment.
- Death.

would include descriptions of violent seizures or the deliberate warming of a thermometer to simulate high fever. Once the child is hospitalized, the adult may introduce fecal matter or other substances into the child's IV to actualize the stated symptoms.

The perpetrator of this type of child abuse is usually an individual who has sophisticated knowledge of medical symptoms and appears to be a loving, caring, dedicated, and attentive adult caregiver. In order to satisfy the adult's own need for attention, the adult will put the child's health and well being at risk. Children abused through Munchausen's by Proxy can have long-term physical and psychological damage from unnecessary medical procedures. Death of the child, while not intentional on the part of the adult, is a frequent result.

Osteogenesis Imperfecta (OI)

While child abuse and neglect are serious problems that need to be handled appropriately, the health care provider should be aware that a condition known as osteogenesis imperfecta frequently mimics some of the signs of child physical abuse. Osteogenesis imperfecta is an inherited condition characterized by abnormally brittle bones that are subject to fracture. **Osteogenesis imperfecta congenital** occurs during intrauterine life, and the infant is born with deformities, while in **osteogenesis imperfecta tarda**, fractures start to occur when the child begins to walk.

The similarities to child physical abuse include:

- The appearance that the child has been traumatized.
- Unlikely or unsatisfactory explanations of how the fracture occurred. The guardian may have no idea how the fracture(s) happened and can only speculate; X rays may reveal old fractures in various stages of healing. Some fractures may not have been noticed; consequently, the fractures may be undiagnosed and untreated.
- Evidence of bruising.
- Varied types of fractures.
- On X ray, the bones appear to be normal.

While similarities exist, there are also some important differences from child physical abuse that the medical professional needs to be able to identify. These differences include:

- Blue sclera; OI is usually attended by a blue coloration of the sclera (whites of the eyes), called Lobstein's disease.
- The skull may be an inverted triangular shape.

- The child may be of small stature.
- Excessive mobility of the joints.
- Thin, fragile skin.
- Excessive sweating.
- There may be little soft tissue damage associated with the fracture.
- Crush fractures of the vertebrae.
- X rays that reveal wormian bones (small, irregular bones in the course of the cranial sutures).
- Discolored teeth that break easily.
- Sometimes OI is accompanied by otosclerotic deafness (van der Hoeve's syndrome).

Few patients with osteogenesis imperfecta will exhibit all of the identified abnormalities. Some patients show none of the classical signs of OI, and some children appear outwardly normal in every way. Osteogenesis imperfecta is diagnosed through a skin biopsy. It takes approximately three months to obtain test results.

Sudden Infant Death Syndrome (SIDS)

Sudden infant death syndrome is the sudden and unexpected death of an apparently healthy infant that cannot be attributed to a specific known cause. In the United States, between 7,000–10,000 infants die of SIDS each year. SIDS typically occurs between birth to 9 months of age, with the highest incidence occurring between 3–5 months of age. After the first week of life, it is the leading cause of death in 1-year-olds.

Demographic studies indicate that SIDS occurs throughout the world, affects males slightly more than females, affects non-Caucasians slightly more than Caucasians, and occurs more frequently during the winter months.

Infants most at risk for developing SIDS may have been born prematurely, or may have a history of apnea due to a seizure disorder or hyaline membrane disease. A family history of SIDS, particularly among siblings, with or without apnea, is also considered a risk factor.

In order to assist in distinguishing between victims of child abuse or neglect and SIDS, the medical professional should be aware of the characteristics presented in Table 16-4.

The medical professional may initially suspect SIDS when the identifying characteristics appear to be accurate, and if a parent or caregiver indicates that the infant was well and healthy when put to sleep.

In cases where sudden infant death syndrome is a possibility, there are more victims than the infant who has died. Many misconceptions about SIDS and its

---

Table 16-4   Characteristics of SIDS Infant

- Exhibits no external signs of injury.
- Exhibits the natural appearance of a deceased infant, including:
  - Lividity, a skin discoloration as from venous congestion or the settling of blood in the body.
  - Frothy discharge from the nose and/or mouth.
  - Small marks, like diaper rash, that may appear more severe.
  - Rigor mortis takes place quickly in infants, approximately 3 hours.
  - There may be purple markings on the head and face.
  - The infant appears to be well developed, yet may be small for its age.
  - Other children in the family appear to be normal and healthy.

---

cause give rise to feelings of guilt or anger on the part of the parents or care-givers, making handling a heartbreaking situation much more difficult. It is important to realize that individuals experiencing grief may try to rationalize what part they may have played in the infant's death and may blame themselves for their loss. Among these misconceptions are ideas that lack of breastfeeding, use of oral contraceptives, or exposure to fluoridation or X rays may have contributed to the infant's death. These are misconceptions, and the professional will need to offer psychological first aid until more complete and thorough assistance or counseling can be obtained.

Behavioral Characteristics of the Abused Child

A child who is being abused may exhibit certain behavioral characteristics inconsistent with the child's age or developmental stage.

Behavioral Indicators of the Abused Child

The child may:

- Be wary of adult contact.
- Be apprehensive or upset when other children cry.
- Exhibit behavior extremes. The child may be extremely aggressive, demanding, or hateful or may be withdrawn, overly compliant, or passive.
- Appear frightened of the caregiver.
- Wear long sleeves or long pants in hot weather to cover bruises.
- Be too eager to please.

- Cringe or jump at sudden movement.
- Show a reversal in roles. The child may parent the parent or act inappropriately adult-like and responsible.
- Verbally report abuse.
- Exhibit developmental lags and fall behind in language development, social skills, motor skills, or toilet training.

While there are many physical indicators of child physical abuse that the health care provider should be aware of, the professional should also be able to recognize those behavioral characteristics in the caregiver that may indicate a possible abusive situation. Combined with inappropriate explanations for the cause of injuries, the health care professional can determine cause for concern and reporting.

Behavioral Indicators of the Abusive Caregiver

Behavioral indicators of the caregiver include:

- Using harsh discipline that is inappropriate to the child's age, behavior, condition, or developmental stage.
- Attempt to conceal or hide the child's injury.
- Give inappropriate or inconsistent explanations as to the cause of the child's injury.
- Become defensive, or refuse to answer questions about the child's injury.

Child Physical Neglect

Child neglect involves inattention to the basic needs of the child. This means that the child is lacking supervision, appropriate food, clothing, shelter, and/or medical attention, and may be exposed to an unhealthy physical environment as well as inappropriate or inadequate hygiene (see Figure 16-5). While physical abuse tends to be episodic, true neglect tends to be chronic, or ongoing. There are many influences—an illness in the family or differences in cultural child-raising practices, for example—that might cause a neglectful situation. It is important for the health care provider to recognize whether or not the child's health, well-being, and development are at risk.

Typical indicators of physical neglect may be seen in lack of supervision, where:

- Very young children are left in the care of other children too young to adequately protect or care for them.

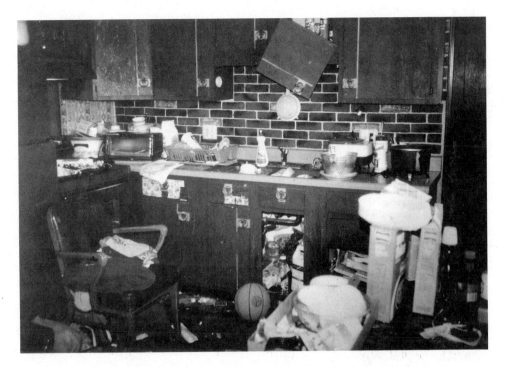

Figure 16-5 An example of physical neglect—an unhealthy physical environment.

- Children are abandoned.
- Children are inadequately supervised over long periods of time or are engaged in dangerous activities.

It is important to use common sense when discussing lack of supervision. While it may be acceptable to leave a mature 10-year-old home alone for half an hour to run to the grocery, it would not be acceptable to leave the same child home alone until late into the evening.

Physical Indicators of Neglect

Lack of Adequate Clothing and Good Personal Hygiene may be indicators of neglect, including:

- Children are dressed inappropriately for the weather.
- Children consistently wear clothing that is torn or dirty.
- Children themselves are consistently dirty or unbathed.
- Children have persistent skin disorders, such as diaper rash or dermatological problems consistent with poor hygiene.

- There is lack of medical or dental care, including lack of provision of necessary health aids.

Lack of Adequate Nutrition could also be a sign of neglect and may include:

- Children who are not provided a sufficient amount of food or are not provided an appropriate quality of nutrition.
- Children who fall 3–4 standard deviations below the normal height or weight for their age, with no acceptable physiological explanation.

Behavioral Indicators of the Neglected Child

Children who are being neglected frequently exhibit behavioral characteristics that can be a clue indicating lack of care. Those behaviors include:

- Constantly complaining of hunger.
- Begging or stealing food.
- Constant fatigue or listlessness.
- Developmental lags.
- Alcohol or other drug abuse.
- Frequent absences from school.
- Delinquency, such as theft or vandalism.
- Reports of being left alone or abandoned.

Behavioral Indicators of the Negligent Caregiver

As with the physical abuse of children, caregivers neglecting the children in their care also frequently exhibit characteristic behaviors that can act as a signal for the health care professional to suspect neglect. Those behaviors include expecting children to care for themselves at an early age, maintaining a chaotic home life, or exhibiting a sense of futility or apathy. Alcohol or other drug abuse can also be an influencing factor in neglect.

Sexual Abuse of the Child

Sexual abuse includes any contact or interaction between a child and an adult that takes place for the sexual stimulation or gratification of the adult. Sexual abuse can be committed by a person under the age of 18 when that person is significantly older than the child or is in a position of power or control over the child. Children from infancy to the teen years have been identified as victims of sexual abuse.

The typical victim of sexual abuse is female. It is important to remember, however, that boys are also victims. Perpetrators of sexual abuse are not always male, either. Women can also commit acts constituting sexual abuse, and adolescents are the perpetrators in at least 20 percent of the reported cases. Sexual abuse is usually committed by someone who is known to the child.

There are both physical and behavioral indicators of child sexual abuse. The physical indicators of sexual abuse (and some of the behavioral indicators) are not normally seen in young children and are difficult or impossible to explain by any other cause. Physical indicators are not always present in children who have been sexually abused. Likewise, some of the behavioral characteristics can be seen in children who are victims of physical or emotional abuse.

There are many types of sexual abuse, and not all involve intercourse. Included are the obvious situations like rape, molestation, prostitution, and incest. However, deviant conduct, child exploitation, child seduction, public indecency, obscene performance, and voyeurism involving a child are also considered to be child sexual abuse.

Physical Indicators of the Sexually Abused Child

The most common physical indicators of child sexual abuse include:

- Any sexually transmitted disease; gonorrheal infection of the throat, genitals, or rectum.
- Pregnancy in a girl under the age of sixteen.
- Pelvic inflammatory disease (PID).
- Foreign material in the bladder, rectum, urethra, or vagina.
- Recurrent urinary tract infections without a physiological basis.
- Bruised or dilated genitals or rectum.
- Difficulty or pain in walking and/or sitting.
- Stained or bloody underclothing.

Behavioral Indicators of the Sexually Abused Child

Behaviors of the child who is being sexually abused might include:

- Seductive behavior, advanced sexual knowledge for the child's age, promiscuity, or prostitution.
- Drawing pictures of people showing genitals (for very young ages and under most circumstances, this behavior would be inappropriate).
- Sexually abusing another child.
- Self-destructive behavior. Even young children can attempt suicide.

- Sleep disorders.
- Noticeable changes in behavior, such as regression, withdrawal, inability to concentrate.
- Taking frequent baths or showers, especially after seeing a particular person.
- Unwillingness to change clothing for physical education classes or to participate in those classes.
- Precocious sex play or compulsive masturbation.
- Expressing fear of a particular person or place.
- Exhibition of behavior extremes.
- Expression of general feelings of shame or guilt.
- Manifestation of poor self-esteem.
- Development of an eating disorder.
- Reporting of the abuse.

It is important to note that some of these behaviors are more specific to certain ages than others. Some of these behaviors may also be attributable to other stressors in the child's life. If sexual abuse is suspected, the situation should be reported to the appropriate child protection agency.

Behavioral Indicators of the Sexually Abusive Caregiver

Caregivers also frequently exhibit behaviors that are not typical of a healthy adult-child relationship. The adult may be extremely protective of the child or may be jealous of the child who is the focus of the sexual abuse. The adult may encourage the child to participate in prostitution or engage in sexual activities in the presence of the caregiver. While child sexual abuse is considered unacceptable under any circumstances, it is possible in some cases for the perpetrators to have an unresolved history as a victim of child sexual abuse themselves. Under these circumstances, the individual's ability to recognize behavior that is injurious to the child may be limited.

Emotional Maltreatment

Emotional maltreatment is more difficult to define and recognize than physical abuse or neglect because it leaves no marks on the child or indicators in the child's physical environment. Emotional maltreatment is a pattern of behavior that has both short-term and long-term effects on the child. While physical injuries heal, emotional or psychological injuries may take a lifetime for recovery.

The effects of such maltreatment can handicap a child in dealing with others because loss of self-esteem is a common effect that typically influences social and developmental interaction.

Emotional maltreatment can be of two types. **Emotional neglect** is the failure of the caregiver to provide the child with the affection, support, and guidance necessary to foster healthy personality development. **Emotional abuse** involves a chronic attitude of the caregiver detrimental to the child's emotional development.

Behavioral Indicators of the Emotionally Abused Child

The following are the most common behavioral indicators of child emotional maltreatment. It is important to remember, however, that some of these behaviors can be triggered by situational circumstances or the developmental stage of the child. Young children, for example, become defiant periodically, even in the most nurturing environments. It is part of their developmental process—they are learning where their boundaries have been set and are trying out their increasing language skills. Behavioral indicators of emotional maltreatment include:

- Withdrawal/anti-social behavior.
- Lack of self-esteem.
- Poor relationships with playmates or children of their own age.
- Apathy.
- Habit disorders such as rocking, thumb-sucking, or head banging in an older child.
- Lack of healthy exploration and creativity—the child may not know how to play.
- Sleep problems or frequent nightmares.
- Daytime anxiety and unrealistic fears.
- Defiant behavior.
- Behavior extremes; overly aggressive or passive, exhibiting infantile behavior or adult-like behavior inconsistent with the child's actual age, or the child may be extremely rigid in behaviors or overly impulsive.
- Irrational and persistent fears or hatreds.
- Seems removed from reality, excessive daydreaming, over-fantasizing.
- Suicide attempts.
- Appearing to get pleasure from hurting other children, adults, or pets.
- In infants, a failure to thrive.
- Developmental lags.

Behavioral Indicators of the Emotionally Abusive Caregiver

As with other types of abuse and neglect, caregivers who are being emotionally abusive frequently exhibit certain behaviors that the health care provider may observe. Emotional abuse is not just an isolated incident. It is unrealistic to think that adults will never say a cross word to a child and will have limitless patience. Everyone says hurtful things sometimes, even unintentionally. An abusive individual says or does hurtful things most of the time. Emotionally abusive behaviors on the part of the caregiver include:

- **Rejecting**—The individual may belittle or criticize the child so that the child is made to feel stupid, ugly, or incompetent. The caregiver may treat the child without affection or treat the child differently from other children in the household.

- **Ignoring**—The adult caregiver may take little or no interest in the child or the child's activities, may not speak to the child very much or be concerned about the child's problems, and may not participate in routine activities with the child.

- **Isolating**—The child may be prevented from participating in social activities consistent with the child's age, or may be prevented from forming any friendships or attachments.

- **Terrorizing**—Children can be terrorized in many different ways, all of which may damage their self-esteem, self-image, and feelings of security. Blaming the child for things they have no control over, using the child as a scapegoat for problems or mishaps, and ridiculing or shaming the child, especially in front of friends, have a negative effect on the child. Terrorizing can also include threatening the child's health and safety, threatening the health and safety of pets, or destroying the child's possessions.

- **Corrupting**—Children need to learn what is right and wrong by adult example and teaching, which also means that the child can be taught socially deviant behavior. The caregiver may demand or reward aggression, encourage stealing or other delinquent acts, or encourage sexually precocious behavior.

False Reporting

A child's report or admission of abuse or neglect must always be taken seriously. According to the National Committee for the Prevention of Child Abuse, all available information suggests that false reports are a rare occurrence. More adults make false reports than children do. Frequently, false reports made by adults come from anonymous sources or are made during child-custody disputes. One should not disregard a child's report based simply on custody disagreements. Any time there is a "reason to believe" that abuse or neglect is taking place, a report must be made to the appropriate agency.

State agencies for reporting child abuse and neglect are included in Appendix D.

Summary

The health care provider comes into contact with a wide range of individuals every day. Some of those contacts will be with victims of different forms of abuse and/or neglect. When it is suspected that children are being abused or neglected, it is the health care professional's responsibility to report that concern to the appropriate agency so that if a problem does exist, the family will be able to get some assistance in resolving the situation in a positive manner.

Abuse and neglect cut across all social, ethnic, racial, age, gender, religious, and economic boundaries. Anyone can be a victim, and anyone can be a perpetrator of abuse. It is important for the skilled health care provider to be able to recognize both physical and behavioral signs and symptoms associated with abuse and neglect, and to be able to identify and follow designated protocol for reporting to the appropriate state agency.

Review Questions

1. Identify the characteristics of children at risk for becoming abused or neglected.
2. Child abuse and neglect cause some generalized effects on children, regardless of the type of abuse or neglect. Identify those effects.
3. Define physical abuse, and give examples of specific indicators, including bruising, burns, fractures, and lacerations.
4. Describe how to date bruises.
5. Define Shaken Baby Syndrome.
6. Define Munchausen's Syndrome by Proxy.
7. Describe osteogenesis imperfecta, and explain how it is sometimes confused with child physical abuse.
8. Describe SIDS.
9. Describe the behavioral characteristics typical of children who are being physically abused.
10. Define physical neglect.

11. List the behavioral characteristics typical of children who are being physically neglected.
12. Define sexual abuse, and list the different forms of sexual abuse.
13. List the most common indicators of child sexual abuse.
14. List the behaviors that may be exhibited by the child who is being sexually abused.
15. What is the difference between emotional abuse and emotional neglect?
16. Describe the behavioral characteristics that a child who is being emotionally abused or neglected might exhibit.
17. Describe the behaviors of the caregiver that are indicative of emotional maltreatment.
18. How common is false reporting?

CHAPTER 17

Adult Victims of Abuse

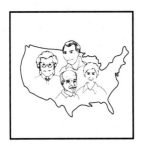

Objectives

After completing this chapter the learner should be able to:

1. Identify at least 3 societal perceptions that contribute to the problem of adult abuse. Students should be able to explain why these are contributing factors.
2. Define rape and describe what steps should be taken to assist the victim of this violent crime.
3. Define elder mistreatment.
4. List at least 1 theory for the occurrence of elder abuse.
5. List the 7 types of elder mistreatment.
6. Describe the causes of self-neglect.

Introduction

For decades, various types of abuse have been a routine fact of life for many. Under certain circumstances, everyone has the potential for becoming abusive, and everyone has the potential for becoming a victim of abuse. This chapter discusses adult victims of abuse. The characteristics of individuals who engage in abusive behavior have been covered in Chapter 15, Recognizing Victims of Abuse or Neglect.

Although anyone can become a victim, women and children are the most common targets. The elderly are also frequently victims because they are in a position where they may have difficulty fighting back. This does not mean that men have never been victims of abusive relationships or situations. Statistics have shown, however, that for a variety of reasons, men are not primary targets of physical abuse.

This chapter deals with societal perceptions that often contribute to this problem. It also covers various aspects of the elder mistreatment.

Societal Perceptions

Common societal perceptions include:

- The belief that battered or abused women are uneducated and have few job skills. In reality, the higher level of education a woman has, the more likely she is to be abused. If one partner in a relationship continues to grow intellectually, the other partner may feel like they are losing control unless the couple continues to grow together.

- The perception that only a small percentage of women are battered or abused. Statistically, nearly 2 million women are abused every year, and half of all women encounter some form of abuse at least once during their marriage or long-term relationship.

- The belief that women are beaten because they deserve it. There is no excuse for physical violence or emotional abuse. If assault and battery took place in another type of relationship, it would be viewed immediately as a criminal act.

- The belief that victims can leave the abusive environment. While many communities now have shelters for women and children who are victims of violence, it is not always easy to leave the situation. There is always the concern for financial support and the belief that the children need both parents. There may be threats against the woman's life, or the lives of the children or other family members, the threat of self destruction from the partner, the threat that the children will be taken away, or the fear of starting over—alone. The woman may know little of community supports. She may feel that the abuse is deserved, and may have been raised in an environment where violence was the norm and not the exception.

- The societal perception that middle-class women do not have to deal with domestic violence as frequently as women in the lower socioeconomic groups. Domestic violence cuts across all socioeconomic boundaries. The higher socioeconomic factions do not report the violence as often as other groups.

- The belief that consumption of alcohol is the cause of battering or abuse. Alcohol may reinforce abusive behavior, but it is not the cause. It is, however, the excuse that may be used to justify unacceptable behavior.

- The perception that abusers are always abusive to their partners. Individuals who are abusive are often loving partners much of the time. They are truly apologetic and often affectionate when asking for forgiveness and another chance.

- The belief that an individual who batters or is abusive is that way in all relationships. This is not always the case. Relationships with other members of the family, or with those outside of the family, may be friendly and normal.

The typical symptoms or indicators of adult abuse mirror many of the characteristics of children who have been abused or neglected. When working with a suspected victim of abuse, it is important to know about community supports so that referrals for assistance can be given. Concerns should also be directed to the physician.

Rape

Rape is defined by law as an individual having sexual intercourse with a member of the opposite sex (this varies from state-to-state and may include members of the same sex) when:

- It is against the wishes of the individual and consent has not been given.
- The individual is unaware that intercourse is taking place.
- The individual is not in a position to give consent.

In the United States, 1 woman in 3 will be or has been the victim of rape or attempted rape. Rape is considered to be an act of violence and not an act of passion. It is a means of one person forcing control over another. Women are the primary targets of rape, and women ages 14–22 are most at risk, particularly for date or acquaintance rape. This does not mean that older women or children cannot be victims of sexual assault, nor does it mean that men cannot be victims.

Any time the medical professional is working with a victim of rape, it is important to understand that rape is not the victim's fault. It is a physical assault that leaves physical and emotional injury. The victims may feel that the situation was their fault and may become depressed and withdrawn. They may become fearful of people whom they know as well as people whom they do not know and may not want anyone to touch them or get too close. They may have trouble sleeping or may be restless. In an attempt to forget, they may be unwilling to discuss the rape or even mention it. After a while they may be unable to get on with their life, until the fears are dealt with.

A victim of rape, regardless of age or gender, should be encouraged to get counseling. Many areas have community mental health services, rape counseling centers, and crisis centers that are skilled in helping the victim deal with physical and emotional injuries. Physical injuries may heal, but emotional trauma such as that associated with rape is difficult to deal with alone. Counseling is recommended.

Some states by law do not require the medical office to report rapes; however, victims should be encouraged, not forced, to report the rape to law enforcement authorities. In the event that the professional is assisting a rape victim, it is important that none of the victim's clothing be destroyed because it can be used as evidence.

Elder Mistreatment

While child and spousal abuse have been receiving widespread media and community attention for nearly 3 decades, it was not until the 1970s that elder mistreatment also began to be recognized as a significant problem. The earliest modern reports came out of the United Kingdom, where case reports about "Granny battering" or "Granny bashing" were released. By the end of the 1970s, elder mistreatment was recognized as a problem in the United States as well.

As with other types of abuse or neglect, both the victims and the perpetrator of elder mistreatment span a broad range of age, gender, racial, ethnic, religious, and socioeconomic boundaries. It has been estimated that approximately 10 percent of the elderly (aged 65 and over) are abused and/or neglected in some manner.

The perpetrator of elder mistreatment is frequently the spouse or an adult child of the older person, but informal or paid caregivers may also be involved. Several theories have been developed that may help the health care professional to understand the phenomenon of elder mistreatment.

The family violence theory asserts that violence is a learned behavior and, essentially, "what goes around comes around." Individuals who have been victims of family violence or who have witnessed such violence may deal with their problems in a similar manner. A second theory indicates that alcoholism, drug addiction, or severe emotional problems may hamper the caregiver's ability to provide adequate support to the elderly. Another theory states that medical, functional, or mental disability of elderly persons increases their dependence and vulnerability, consequently increasing their risk for mistreatment. Approximately 80 percent of those individuals over age 65 are taking medication(s) for one or more chronic health problems. The older the person, the more likely the possibility of the development or progression of significant, possibly debilitating, physical and/or mental conditions. The caregiver may also be economically dependent on the older person who needs care, contributing to resentment of the older person and, when combined with other factors, leading to an abusive or neglectful situation.

Other theories target stress as a major contributing factor to the mistreatment. In addition to the normal daily stressors that occur, the "caregiver" also takes on the stress of that particular role. Economic pressures, increasing care needs, and lack of community and family support all add to the stress the caregiver may experience.

There are barriers to understanding the elderly, which may translate in some cases into barriers in identifying mistreatment. Society in general has many misconceptions about the aging process. These misconceptions about aging enable individuals to overlook or "chalk up to getting old" problems or situations that would be handled quickly and efficiently in a younger population. Ageist views of society include a belief that functional decline and fragility are an inevitable result of aging. In fact, however, many of the problems encountered in old age, such as incontinence, impaired mobility, and "failure to thrive" may be due to treatable, organic causes. Problems like confusion or fatigue might be due to inappropriate medications. If these conditions can be treated, older persons can frequently contribute more to their own care.

In a broad sense, elder mistreatment means the violation of any legal or human right that is accorded to all members of society. As with all other age groups, these rights promote the concepts of self-respect and dignity, and include privacy and free speech.

Categories/Types of Elder Mistreatment

Elder mistreatment falls into seven separate categories/types:

1. **Physical Abuse**—This abuse involves any act of violence that may result in pain, injury, impairment, or disease. It includes pushing, hitting, pinching, slapping, biting, burning, striking with an object, force-feeding, improper use of physical restraints, incorrect positioning, sexual assault, or coercion.

2. **Physical Neglect**—Situations involving physical neglect may be characterized by the withholding of health maintenance care, including proper

nutrition or meals, adequate hydration, appropriate physical personal hygiene, or physical therapy. Failure to provide appropriate physical aids such as eyeglasses, hearing aids, dentures, or walkers, or failure to provide proper safety measures, are all included in physical neglect. Suspicion of physical neglect should be aroused if the older person exhibits signs of dehydration or malnutrition that cannot be reasonably explained by illness, decubitus ulcers (see Figure 17-1), poor personal hygiene, or failure to comply with medical regimens without appropriate or reasonable explanation.

3. **Psychological Abuse**—Each individual regardless of age or physical circumstances has the right to be treated with respect. Any conduct that causes mental anguish can be construed as psychological abuse, including isolating the older person from family and friends, threats of punishment or deprivation, intimidation, treating the older person like a young child, verbal berating, or harassment.

4. **Psychological Neglect**—This form of neglect involves failure to provide the elderly person with social stimulation. The elderly person may be left alone for long periods of time, may be ignored or given the "silent treatment," or may be deprived of companionship, changes in routine, or access to news via personal communication, television, radio, or printed materials.

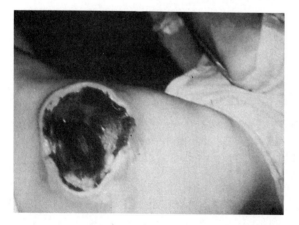

Figure 17-1 Deep (crater) lesion, also known as a decubitus ulcer. (Photo courtesy of Emory University Hospital, Atlanta, Georgia.)

5. **Financial or Material Abuse**—If a caregiver or advisor misuses an elderly individual's income or their resources for the personal or financial gain of the caregiver or advisor, the result is financial abuse. This type of abuse can involve denying the older person a home, or stealing money or possessions. It may also involve coercing the older person to assign durable power of attorney to someone, to make changes in a will, or to sign contracts. Financial abuse is more common with older people because they are more likely to have assets, such as a home, bank accounts, investments, or other valuables.

6. **Financial or Material Neglect**—Financial neglect should be suspected if the elderly person is suffering from substandard care even though adequate financial resources are available to provide an appropriate standard of care. Another indication of possible financial neglect would be an elderly person's confusion or lack of awareness regarding their financial resources, or if assets have been suddenly transferred to another individual without reasonable explanation.

7. **Violation of Personal Rights**—The majority of elderly persons are capable of making reasoned decisions for themselves. They should not be denied the right to use their own judgment and capabilities in providing for their own welfare, needs, and care. Failure to recognize the older person's dignity and autonomy can include:

   ▪ Denying the older individual the right to privacy.

   ▪ Forcible eviction; placement in an alternate facility or nursing home; or denying the person the right to make decisions regarding health care, personal well-being, or other individual matters.

Self-neglect

A variety of circumstances can also contribute to a condition called self-neglect. Self-neglect is the failure or inability of an individual to provide or arrange adequate and appropriate means necessary for personal, physical, medical, mental, and emotional needs. Any adult can suffer from self-neglect. It is a problem in our older population for a variety of reasons, some related to the aging process, some a result of life stresses. Considering all that is necessary to maintain good physical, mental, and emotional health, when circumstances of an individual's life change significantly, it is easy to fall into a pattern of self-neglect.

Stressors that Influence Ability for Self-care

As with any age group, older people are susceptible to a variety of stressors that influence their ability for self-care:

Organic Brain Dysfunction Similar symptoms appear in most organic brain disorders. While these symptoms may be the result of different causes, the symptoms exhibited are related to physical changes in the brain. When behavioral or emotional changes have no identifiable organic cause and are not specifically related to known brain deterioration, the individual suffers from functional mental disorder. These symptoms may be slight or profound, and may come on quite suddenly or develop gradually over a period of time. Functional mental disorders are classified by different types of mental changes, including:

- **Impaired Memory**—Inability to register an event, failure to retain memory of an event, or inability to voluntarily recall a memory.
- **Impaired Intellect**—The individual has trouble understanding facts or ideas, and may have trouble handling even simple mathematical chores or learning something new.
- **Impaired Judgment**—The person may have difficulty comprehending personal situations, and may be unable to make reasoned decisions regarding personal circumstances.
- **Impaired Orientation**—Primarily described as confusion, the individual may have difficulty relating to time, places, or the identity of others.
- **Excessive or Shallow Emotions**—Emotions may shift rapidly, or the individual may overreact or react very little to significant events.

The health care professional should remember that only a small percentage of older people suffer degenerative brain disease or decreased mental functioning. As most people get older, a far larger portion of the elderly population experience "crystalline thinking" or "crystalline intelligence," an increased ability in problem solving rather than decreased mental functioning.

Bereavement As an individual ages, loss of close friends and family becomes increasingly frequent. In any long-term relationship, the individuals left behind after a death typically experience not only a sense of loss, but also a feeling that their own life has lost purpose; they may simply "bide their time" until it is their turn to die. Any significant loss involves a grieving process, and until this is worked through, persons will need support before their own grief recovery and healing can begin. During this process, they may tend to neglect their own good health habits.

Retirement Our population is living longer now than at any other time in history. Many people reach an age where retirement from the typical work environment is either welcomed, perceived as a necessity, or required by government regulations. For some individuals, retirement is a welcome opportunity to do some of the things they did not have time for while employed. For others, it heralds a swift decline in what the person considers their usefulness to society. The way in which a person handles retirement is directly related to health and life circumstances, as well as outside interests. A person who was physically, socially, or creatively active before retirement typically remains so after retirement. Persons whose self-image is linked directly to their job, however, may not know what to do with the time at their disposal in retirement, and may see it as the end. Loss of self-worth and problems with personal identity may develop once work ceases to be part of everyday life. With a sense of loss of purpose or usefulness comes a rise in the tendency for self-neglect.

Depression Everyone sometimes needs solitude, time alone. By nature, however, human beings regardless of age are social beings. When people are isolated by circumstances beyond their control—loss of friends or family, or decreased mobility, for example—depression is a condition that can arise. Symptoms of depression include loss of appetite, fitful sleep, early morning awakening, weight loss, loss of energy and motivation, sometimes even thoughts of suicide. Depression is a natural byproduct of a loss of any kind, whether that loss is of another person or change in personal circumstances. If the depression does not lift, however, the situation could be serious, and a physician should be consulted.

The Body's Warning Signals

Some body changes are inevitable as a person ages, and risk for certain diseases increases as the individual gets older. Not all changes in health are related to the gradual physical decline brought on by aging; consequently, the individual should pay prompt attention to minor disabilities. Many situations can be alleviated or resolved and the individual's level of functioning, whether physical or mental, brought back to a more acceptable level.

Summary

Whether an older person is being abused or neglected by someone else, or whether the circumstances involve self-neglect, the key to assistance is recognizing that a problem situation may exist, and making those concerns known. As a health care provider involved in initial patient contact, you should express these concerns to the treating physician so that clarification of a possible problem can be made, and either referrals or contact with the appropriate community agency can be instituted. Appendix E contains a state-by-state listing of aging and adult protective service agencies that can be used for information or reporting.

Review Questions

1. Describe the term "adult abuse." Be prepared to cite at least one reason for its occurrence.
2. How is rape defined in the textbook? Do you agree with the text? List and discuss 4 reasons for agreeing or disagreeing.
3. You are the Medical Assistant at the clinic when, around 1:00 A.M., a bloody-faced female with torn clothing runs in and says, "I've been raped!" Describe how you would handle this situation. Explain your responses.
4. Describe an individual in your life (without giving names) whom you thought of as you read the information on elder mistreatment. Why did this particular person come to mind?

APPENDIX A

1990 DACUM Analysis of the Medical Assisting Profession

1.0 DISPLAY PROFES-SIONALISM	1.1 Project a Positive Attitude	1.2 Perform within Ethical Boundaries	1.3 Practice Within the Scope of Education Training and Personal Capabilities	1.4 Maintain Confiden-tiality	1.5 Work as a Team Member	1.6 Conduct Oneself in a Courteous and Diplomatic Manner	1.7 Adapt to Change
2.0 COMMUNI-CATE	2.1 Listen and Observe	2.2 Treat All Patients With Empathy and Impartiality	2.3 Adapt Communica-tion to Individuals' Abilities to Understand	2.4 Recognize and Respond to Verbal and Non-verbal Communica-tion	2.5 Serve as Liaison Between Physician and Others	2.6 Evaluate Under-standing of Communi-cation	2.7 Receive, Organize, Prioritize and Transmit Information
3.0 PERFORM ADMINIS-TRATIVE DUTIES	3.1 Perform Basic Secretarial Skills	3.2 Schedule and Monitor Appoint-ments	3.3 Prepare and Maintain Medical Records	3.4 Apply Computer Concepts for Office Procedures	3.5 Perform Medical Transcription	3.6 Locate Resources and Infor-mation for Patients and Employees	3.7 Manage Physician's Professional Schedule and Travel
4.0 PERFORM CLINICAL DUTIES	4.1 Apply Principles of Aseptic Technique and Infection Control	4.2 Take Vital Signs	4.3 Recognize Emergencies	4.4 Perform First Aid and CPR	4.5 Prepare and Maintain Examination and Treatment Area	4.6 Interview and Take Patient History	4.7 Prepare Patients for Procedures
5.0 APPLY LEGAL CONCEPTS TO PRACTICE	5.1 Document Accurately	5.2 Determine Needs for Documen-tation and Reporting	5.3 Use Appropriate Guidelines When Releasing Records or Information	5.4 Follow Established Policy in Initiating or Terminating Medical Treatment	5.5 Dispose of Controlled Substances in Com-pliance With Government Regulations	5.6 Maintain Licenses and Accreditation	5.7 Monitor Legislation Related to Current Healthcare Issues and Practice
6.0 MANAGE THE OFFICE	6.1 Maintain the Physical Plant	6.2 Operate and Maintain Facilities and Equipment Safely	6.3 Inventory Equipment and Supplies	6.4 Evaluate and Recommend Equipment and Supplies for a Practice	6.5 Maintain Liability Coverage	6.6 Exercise Efficient Time Management	Supervise* Personnel
7.0 PROVIDE INSTRUC-TION	7.1 Orient Patients to Office Policies and Procedures	7.2 Instruct Patients With Special Needs	7.3 Teach Patients Methods of Health Promotion and Disease Prevention	7.4 Orient and Train Personnel	Provide* Health Information for Public Use	Supervise* Student Practicums	Conduct* Continuing Education Activities
8.0 MANAGE PRACTICE FINANCES	8.1 Use Manual Bookkeeping Systems	8.2 Implement Current Procedural Terminology and ICD-9 Coding	8.3 Analyze and Use Current Third-Party Guidelines for Reim-bursement	8.4 Manage Accounts Receivable	8.5 Manage Accounts Payable	8.6 Maintain Records for Accounting and Banking Purposes	8.7 Process Employee Payroll

*Denotes advanced-level skills. The medical assistant should be able to perform all other skills after completing a CAHEA-accred-ited program and starting a first job.

1.8 Show Initiative and Responsibility	1.9 Promote the Profession	Enhance* Skills Through Continuing Education					
2.8 Use Proper Telephone Technique	**2.9 Interview Effectively**	**2.10 Use Medical Terminology Appropriately**	2.11 Compose Written Communication Using Correct Grammar, Spelling and Format	Develop* and Conduct Public Relations Activities Market Professional Services			
4.8 Assist Physician With Examinations and Treatment	4.9 Use Quality Control	4.10 Collect and Process Specimens	4.11 Perform Selected Tests That Assist With Diagnosis and Treatment	4.12 Screen and Follow-up Patient Test Results	4.13 Prepare and Administer Medications as Directed by Physician	**4.14 Maintain Medication Records**	**Respond* to Medical Emergencies**
Develop* and Maintain Policy and Procedure Manuals	Establish* Risk Management Protocol for the Practice						
Develop* Job Descriptions	Interview* and Recommend New Personnel	Negotiate* Leases and Prices for Equipment and Supply Contracts					
Develop* Educational Materials							
Manage* Personnel Benefits and Records							

Reprinted with permission. The American Association of Medical Assistants, Inc. 20 North Wacker Drive, Chicago, Illinois 60606 312-899-1500 Toll free 800-228-2262

APPENDIX B

OSHA'S Blood-Borne Pathogen and Universal Precaution Guidelines (Effective March 6, 1992)* (*Federal Register,* December 6, 1991)

To whom does it apply?

All health care workers, service employees, and so on, who may be occupationally exposed to blood or other potentially infectious materials.

Why was the rule established?

To reduce occupational exposure of employees and to reduce workplace exposures to blood-borne pathogens.

Definitions

Blood means human blood, human blood components, and products made from human blood.

Blood-borne Pathogens means pathogenic microorganisms that are present in human blood and can cause disease in humans. These pathogens include, but are not limited to, hepatitis-B virus (HBV) and human immunodeficiency virus (HIV).

*Adapted from Occupational Exposure to Blood Borne Pathogen, U.S. Department of Labor, OSHA, OSHA pamphlet no. 3127.

Clinical Laboratory means a workplace where diagnostic or other screening procedures are performed on blood or other potentially infectious materials.

Contaminated means the presence or the reasonably anticipated presence of blood or other potentially infectious materials on an item or surface.

Contaminated Laundry means laundry that has been soiled with blood or other potentially infectious materials or may contain sharps.

Contaminated Sharps means any contaminated object that can penetrate the skin including, but not limited to, needles, scalpels, broken glass, broken capillary tubes, and exposed ends of dental wires.

Decontamination means the use of physical or chemical means to remove, inactivate, or destroy blood-borne pathogens on a surface or item to the point where they are not longer capable of transmitting infectious particles, and the surface or item is rendered safe for handling, use, or disposal.

Exposure Controls means controls (that is, sharps disposal containers, self-sheathing needles) that isolate or remove the blood-borne pathogen hazard from the workplace.

Exposure Incident means a specific eye, mouth, or other mucous membrane, non-intact skin, or parenteral contact with blood or other potentially infectious materials that results from the performance of an employee's duties.

Handwashing Facilities means a facility providing an adequate supply of running potable water, soap, and single-use towels or hot-air drying machines.

Occupational Exposure means reasonably anticipated skin, eye, mucous membrane, or parenteral contact with blood or other potentially infectious materials that may result from the performance of an employee's duties.

Universal Precautions is an approach to infection control. According to the concept of Universal Precautions, all human blood and certain human body fluids are treated as if known to be infectious for HIV, HBV, and other blood-borne pathogens.

The exposure control plan:

1. The employer must develop a written control plan, citing who may be exposed and how, how to evaluate exposure incidents, and a schedule for implementing the standards.
2. The plan must be reviewed and updated annually.
3. All employees must be given information and training at no cost to the employee at their initial hire and annually thereafter.
4. Hepatitis-B vaccination must be made available to all employees at no cost to them within 10 days of initial hire. Employees who decline the service will sign a declination acknowledging continued risk of exposure.

5. Universal precautions must be practiced by all employees, whereby *all* human blood and human body fluids are considered infectious for HIV, HBV, or other blood-borne pathogens.

6. Methods of control include:

   a. Establish engineering control to minimize hazards and reduce employee exposure—puncture-resistant containers to hold sharps, self-sheathing needles, resuscitation bags, and ventilation bags.

   b. Establish workplace controls, including restrictions for eating, drinking, smoking, applying cosmetics or lip balm, handling contact lenses, prohibition of mouth pipetting, standards for food storage, use of handwashing facilities, decontamination of equipment, frequent handwashing, even after removal of rubber gloves, and prohibiting bending, breaking, or recapping needles.

   c. Use personal protective equipment to prevent exposure or contamination, including gloves, gowns, lab coats, face shield, masks, and eye protection that is not permeable to blood or other potentially hazardous infectious materials. Such protection may not be able to pass through protective covering onto street clothes, undergarments, skin, eyes, mouth, and so on.

   d. Employer must provide personal protective equipment at no cost to the employee, and the employee must wear this equipment whenever occupational exposure may occur.

   e. Employer must ensure that employees remove all protective equipment before leaving work area and after it becomes contaminated.

   f. Employer must provide laundry service for cleaning of personal protective equipment and disposal of contaminated equipment.

   g. Employer must ensure that employees wear all personal protective clothing and gear whenever the potential for contamination exists and see that disposable gloves are not washed for reuse.

7. Employer must maintain a clean work environment for employees and establish appropriate decontamination methods for employees to follow. Cleaning standards will apply to the environment, equipment, and work spaces. Spills must be cleaned as follows:

   a. Use tongs, dustpan, and so on to pick up broken glass.

   b. Place contaminated glass in sharps container.

   c. Spray area with 10 percent bleach solution (10 parts water to 1 part bleach), then clean with paper towels.

   d. Discard all contaminated cleaning rags in a biohazards container.

8. Label all containers holding biological materials with the fluorescent orange warning labels. Make sure the warning label is readily visible on all collection containers designated to hold contaminated or infectious waste or materials for use. The biohazard label is shown.

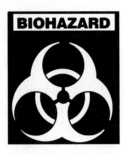

Essentials for laboratory workers:

1. Gloves must be worn at all times when handling all body fluid material.
2. Sharps as well as broken glass must be disposed of in hard-walled sharps containers. Such containers will be strategically placed and readily available for use.
3. Employers must provide nonpermeable protective clothing for those at risk of contamination by potentially hazardous body fluids.
4. Employers must make available hepatitis-B vaccinations at no cost to the employee. Employees may decline but are required to sign a waiver of liability. Employees do have the right to request the vaccination at a later date without cost to them.
5. Employers must provide education and training for their employees.
6. To clean a biohazardous spill, a 3–10 percent bleach solution is poured over the site, allowed to sit, and then cleaned up with disposable towels.
7. Spills on instrumentation are also cleaned with bleach. Equipment sent for repair will be sprayed with a disinfectant bleach before being serviced.
8. Biohazardous trash will be properly disposed of according to weight and volume generated by a facility. Generally, biohazardous waste generated under 50 pounds is exempt from removal by a biohazardous waste management company.
9. Clothing worn on duty by health care personnel will not be worn outside the workplace, even to and from work.

APPENDIX C

Frequently Used
Telephone Numbers

This form can be cut down to a size suitable for taping next to the home telephone. Use the extra lines for the phone numbers of people who are called frequently or who need to be reached in a hurry.

If you live outside the city limits, be certain to check on what fire department to call, and whether to call the city police, state police, or county sheriff for assistance. Write down your address and telephone number. In an emergency, many people may not think clearly, and a delay in assistance could result in a life or death situation. A place for your address is provided.

A version of this form or the form shown in Figure 3-2 can also be used in the medical office. A form with current numbers should be placed near each office phone.

FREQUENTLY USED TELEPHONE NUMBERS	
1. POLICE	
2. FIRE	
3. AMBULANCE	
4. POISON INFORMATION	
5. EMERGENCY	
6. Family Physician (ofc.)	
(home)	
Hospital	
7. Personal Physician (ofc.)	
(home)	
8. Pediatrician (ofc.)	
(home)	
9. Pediatrics Center	
10. Dentist	
11. Optometrist	
12. Time	
13. School	
14. Neighbor for emergency	
Babysitters	
Other	
Designated Relative	
YOUR NAME	
YOUR ADDRESS	
YOUR PHONE #	

APPENDIX D

State Agencies for Reporting Child Abuse and Neglect

Alabama
Department of Human Resources
Montgomery, AL
205 242-9500

Alaska
Local Office of Family and Youth
Services
Statewide 24-hour hot line:
800 478-4444

Arizona
Arizona Department of Economic
Security
(32 regional offices of child protection
services; each has 24-hour hot line)
Phoenix hot line: 800 541-5781

Arkansas
Department of Human Services
Little Rock, AR
800 482-5964

California
Department of Social Services

Office of Child Protective Services
916 657-2030

Colorado
County Office of Department of Social
Services
Denver County: 24-hour hot line:
303 727-3000
Other counties: Call sheriff's office

Connecticut
Department of Human Resources;
Department of Children and Youth
Services
Hartford, CT
203 566-3661 or
800 842-2288; 24-hour hot
line will refer to regional
offices.

Delaware
Department of Services for Children,
Youth & Their Families
Child Protective Services
Wilmington, DE

302 577-2163 or
24-hour hot line: 800 292-9582

District of Columbia
DC Police Department Youth Division
Washington, DC
To report child abuse: 202 576-6762
To report child neglect: 202 727-0995

Florida
Florida Abuse Registry
800 962-2873 (904 487-2625)

Georgia
Department of Human Resources
Child Protective & Placement Services
Atlanta, GA
404 894-5672

Hawaii
Department of Social Services
24-hour hot line: 808 832-5300
Or for information and referral to
regional Dept. of Health Office call
208 334-5700

Illinois
Department of Children and Family
Services
Springfield, IL
217 785-4010
Or 24-hour hot line for
reporting and parents under stress
800 252-2873

Indiana
Indiana Family and Social Services
317 232-4431
Or hot line:
800 562-2407

Iowa
Local Office of Department of Human
Services

Or call state hot line:
800 362-2178

Kansas
Department of Social and Rehabilitative
Services
913 296-4657
Or Department of Social and
Rehabilitative Services
24-hour hot line:
800 922-5330

Kentucky
Local Department for Social Services
Or statewide hot line: 800 752-6200
In Jefferson County call: 502 581-6184
Parents Anonymous: 800 432-9251

Louisiana
Regional Offices of Child Protection
Services
Or call 24-hour hot line: 504 925-4571

Maine
Department of Human Services
Childrens' Emergency Services
207 289-2983
After hours: 800 452-1999 (24-hour)

Maryland
County Office of Department of Social
Services
Each office has 24-hour hot line
Baltimore City hot line:
301 361-2235

Massachusetts
Information packet for
mandated reporters available through
Department of Social Services
Boston, MA
617 727-0900 (x573)
Make reports to area office of

Department of Social Services where
child is resident.
24-hour state hot line:
800 792-5200

Michigan
Each county protective service
(under Department of Social
Services) 24-hour hot line or
Private hot line run by GATEWAYS
can direct to county offices and
provide information:
800 942-4357

Minnesota
County Office of Department of
Human Services
Each office has 24-hour hot line

Mississippi
Department of Human Services
601 354-6659
Or 24-hour
hot line: 800 222-8000

Missouri
Department of Social Services
Child Abuse and Neglect
Jefferson City, MO
314 751-3448
Parental Stress Helpline: 800 367-2543
Reporting: 800 392-3738 (24-hour)

Montana
Department of Family Services
Child Abuse & Neglect Program
Helena, MT
406 444-5900
Or 800 332-6100 (24-hour)

Nebraska
Information:
Department of Social Services-Child
Protective Services
Lincoln, NE

402 471-7000
Reporting:
800 652-1999 (24-hour)

Nevada
Information:
Department of Human Resources
Division of Child and Family Services
Carson City, NV
702 687-5982
Reporting:
Local child protection agency
Or 800 992-5757 (all areas
except Clark County)
702 399-0081 (Clark County)

New Hampshire
Information:
Department of Health and
Welfare Division for Children and
Youth Services
Concord, NH
603 271-4451
Reporting:
800 562-2340 (eastern area)
800 624-9701 (western area)
800 458-5542 (central and northern
areas)
800 852-3388 (24-hour helpline)

New Jersey
Information:
Division of Youth and Family Services
Trenton, NJ
Reporting:
800 792-8610 (24-hour)

New Mexico
Department of Human Services
Social Services Division
Santa Fe, NM
505 827-8400
Or 800 432-6217 (24-hour information
and referral)

New York
Information:
Department of Social Services
Division of Family and Child Services
Albany, NY
518 474-9003 (public information)
Reporting:
800 342-3720 (24-hour)

North Carolina
Information:
Department of Human Resources
Child Protective Service Unit
Raleigh, NC
919 733-2580
Reporting:
Department of Social Services
800 662-7030 (helpline)

North Dakota
Information:
Department of Human Services
Child Abuse and Neglect
Bismarck, ND
701 224-2316
Reporting:
County Social Services

Ohio
Department of Human Services
Child Protective Services Unit
Bureau of Children Services
Columbus, OH
614 466-9824

Oklahoma
Information:
Department of Human Services
Division of Child Welfare
Oklahoma City, OK
405 521-2283
Reporting: 800 522-3511
(24-hour, all areas except Oklahoma
County)

800 841-0800 (24-hour, Oklahoma
County)

Oregon
Information:
Department of Human Resources
Childrens' Services Division
Salem, OR
503 378-4722
Reporting:
County Child Protective Services
Or 503 378-4722

Pennsylvania
Department of Public Welfare
Child Abuse Central Registry
Harrisburg, PA
717 783-8744 or
800 932-0313 (24-hour reporting and
information)

Puerto Rico
Information:
Department of Social Services
Family Services
Santurce, PR
809 724-0303 or 809 723-2127
Reporting: 809 724-1333 (24-hour)

Rhode Island
Information:
Department of Children, Youth, and
Families
Providence, RI
401 457-4708
Reporting: 800 742-4453 (24-hour
reporting and information)

South Carolina
Department of Social Services
Division of Child Protective and
Preventive Services
Columbia, SC
803 734-5670

Tennessee
Department of Human Services
Child Protective Services
Nashville, TN
615 741-5927
After business hours, contact local
sheriff's department

Texas
Information:
Department of Human Services
Childrens' Protective Services
Austin, TX
512 834-0034
Reporting:
800 252-5400 (24-hour)

Utah
Information:
Department of Human Services
Child Abuse
Salt Lake City, UT
801 538-4171
Reporting: 800
678-9399 (24-hour)
801 487-9811 (24-hour
investigation line)

Vermont
Department of Social and
Rehabilitation Services
Division of Social Services
Waterbury, VT
802 241-2131
Emergency/after hours: 800 356-6552

Virginia
Information:
Department of Social Services
Child Protective Services Unit
Richmond, VA
804 662-9081
Reporting: 800 552-7096 (24-hour
within Virginia)

804 662-9084 (24-hour from out of
state)

Washington
Information:
Social and Health Services
Childrens' Protective Services
Olympia, WA
206 753-7002
Reporting: 800 562-5624 (24-hour)

West Virginia
Information:
Department of Health and Human
Resources
Office of Social Services
Charleston, WV
304 348-7980
Reporting: 800 352-6513 (24-hour)

Wisconsin
Department of Health and Social
Services
Office of Child Abuse and Neglect
Madison, WI
608 266-3036

Wyoming
Information:
Department of Family Services
Youth Services Division
Cheyenne, WY
307 777-7150
Reporting: Local county sheriff or
police for oncall social worker

**National Child Abuse Hot
Line (Child Help USA):**
800 422-4453

APPENDIX E

State Aging and Adult Protective Service Agencies

Alabama
Elder Abuse Hotline
In-State: 800 458-7214
Commission on Aging
Montgomery, AL
205 242-5743

Director
Adult Services Division
Department of Human Resources
Montgomery, AL
205 242-1350

Alaska
Older Alaskans Commission
Department of Administration
Juneau, AK
907 465-3250

  Or

Adult Protective Services
Division of Family & Youth Services
Department of Health and Social
Services
Juneau, AK
907 465-2145

Arizona
Aging and Adult Administration
Department of Economic Security
Phoenix, AZ
602 542-4446

Arkansas
Elder Abuse Hotline
In-State: 800 482-8049 or
922-5330
Division of Aging and Adult Services
Department of Human Services
Little Rock, AR
501 682-2441

California
Department of Aging
Sacramento, CA
916 322-5290

  Or

Adult Services Bureau
Department of Social Services
Adult and Family Services
Sacramento, CA
916 657-2186

Colorado
Aging and Adult Services
Department of Social Services
Denver, CO
303 866-3851 or 303 866-5910

Connecticut
Department of Aging
Hartford, CT
203 566-3238

Or

Department of Human Resources
Hartford, CT
203 566-3117

Delaware
Division on Aging
Department of Health and Social
Services
New Castle, DE
302 577-4791

District of Columbia
Office on Aging
Washington, DC
202 724-5626

Or

Family Services Administration
Department of Human Services
Washington, DC
202 727-0113

Florida
Elder Abuse Hotline
In-State: 800 96-ABUSE
Department of Elder Affairs
Tallahassee, FL
904 922-5297

Or

Aging and Adult Services
Department of Health & Rehabilitative

Services
Tallahassee, FL
904 488-2650

Georgia
Office of Aging
Atlanta, GA
404 894-5333

Or

Division of Family & Children Services
Department of Human Resources
Atlanta, GA
404 894-4440

Hawaii
Executive Office on Aging
Office of the Governor
Honolulu, HI
808 586-0100

Or

Adult Services Department of Human
Services
Honolulu, HI
808 548-5902

Idaho
Office on Aging
Boise, ID
208 334-3833

Or

Bureau of Adult Services
Department of Health and Welfare
Boise, ID
208 334-5531

Illinois
Elder Abuse Hotline: 800 252-8966
Department on Aging
Springfield, IL
217 785-2870

Indiana
Adult Abuse Hotline
In-State: 800 992-6978
Bureau of Aging/In-Home Services
Indianapolis, IN
317 232-7020

Or

Department of Human Services
Indianapolis, IN
317 232-1750

Iowa
Elder Abuse Hotline
In-State: 800 362-2178
Department of Elder Affairs
Des Moines, IA
515 281-5187

Or

Bureau of Adult, Children, & Family
Services
Des Moines, IA
515 281-6219

Kansas
Department on Aging
Topeka, KS
913 296-4986

Or

Adult Abuse Program
Department of Social & Rehabilitative
Services
Topeka, KS
913 296-2575

Kentucky
Division of Aging Services
Cabinet for Human Resources
Frankfort, KY
502 564-6930

Or

Adult Services
Division of Family Services
Department of Social Services
Frankfort, KY
502 564-7043

Louisiana
Office of Elderly Affairs
Baton Rouge, LA
504 925-1700

Or

Division of Children, Youth & Family
Services
Department of Social Services
Baton Rouge, LA
504 342-9931

Maine
Elder Abuse Hotline
In-State: 800 442-1999
Bureau of Elder & Adult Services
Department of Human Services
Augusta, ME
207 624-5335

Maryland
Office on Aging
Baltimore, MD
410 225-1100

Or

Adult Protective Services
Department of Human Resources
Baltimore, MD
410 333-0161

Massachusetts
Elder Abuse Hotline
In-State: 800 922-2275
Executive Office of Elder Affairs
Boston, MA
617 727-7750

Or

Protective Services
Executive Office of Elder Affairs
Boston, MA
617 727-7750 Ext 302

Michigan
Office of Services to the Aging
Lansing, MI
517 373-8230

Or

Office of Adult and Employment
Services
Department of Social Services
Lansing, MI
517 373-2869

Minnesota
Elder Abuse Hotline
In-State: 800 652-9747
Board on Aging
St. Paul, MN
612 296-2770

Or

Adult Protection Consultant
Aging and Adult Services
St. Paul, MN
612 296-4019

Mississippi
Elder Abuse Hotline
In-State: 800 354-6347
Council on Aging
Division of Aging and Adult Services
Jackson, MS
601 949-2070

Or

Adult Protection Services
Department of Human Services
Jackson, MS
601 354-6631

Missouri
Elder Abuse Hotline
In-State: 800 392-0210
Division on Aging
Department of Social Services
Jefferson City, MO
314 751-3082

Montana
The Governor's Office on Aging
Helena, MT
406 444-3111

Or

Adult Protective Services
Department of Family Services
Helena, MT
406 444-5900

Nebraska
Elder Abuse Hotline
In-State: 800 652-1999
Department on Aging
Lincoln, NE
402 471-2306

Or

Special Services for Children and Adults
Medical Services Division
Department of Social Services
Lincoln, NE
402 471-9345

Nevada
Division for Aging Services
Department of Human Resources
Las Vegas, NV
702 486-3545

Or

Adult Protective Services
Department of Human Resources
Carson City, NV
702 687-4588

New Hampshire
Elder Abuse Hotline
In-State: 800 852-3345
Division of Elderly & Adult Services
Concord, NH
603 271-4680

New Jersey
Elder Abuse Hotline
In-State: 800 792-8820
Division on Aging
Department of Community Affairs
Trenton, NJ
609 292-4833

Or

Adult Protective Services
Division of Youth and
Family Services
Department of Human Services
Trenton, NJ
609 292-6726

New Mexico
Elder Abuse Hotline
In-State: 800 432-6217
State Agency on Aging
Santa Fe, NM
505 827-7640

Or

Adult Services Bureau
Social Services Division
Human Services Department
Santa Fe, NM
505 827-8402

New York
Office for the Aging
Albany, NY
518 474-4425

Or

Bureau of Community Services
State Department of Social Services
Albany, NY
518 432-2980

North Carolina
Elder Abuse Hotline
In-State: 800 662-7030
Division of Aging
Raleigh, NC
919 733-3983

Or

Adult and Family Services
Division of Social Services
Department of Human Resources
Raleigh, NC
919 733-3818

North Dakota
Aging Services Division
Department of Human Services
Bismarck, ND
701 224-2577

Ohio
Elder Abuse Hotline
In-State: 800 686-1581
Department of Aging
Columbus, OH
614 466-5500

Or

Bureau of Adult Services
Division of Adult &
Child Care Services
Department of Human Services
Columbus, OH
614 466-0995

Oklahoma
Elder Abuse Hotline
In-State: 800 522-3511

Aging Services Division
Department of Human Services
Oklahoma City, OK
405 521-2327

Or

Adult Protective Services
Aging Services Division
Department of Human Services
Oklahoma City, OK
405 521-3660

Oregon
Elder Abuse Hotline
In-State: 800 232-3020
Senior and Disabled Services Division
Salem, OR
503 378-4728

Or

Abuse and Protective Services
Senior Services Division
Department of Human Resources
Salem, OR
503 378-3751

Pennsylvania
Fraud and Abuse Hotline
In-State: 800 992-2433
Department of Aging
Harrisburg, PA
717 783-1550 or 717 783-6007

Puerto Rico
Governor's Office for Elderly Affairs
Santurce, PR
809 721-5710

Or

Services to Adults
Department of Social Services
Santurce, PR
809 723-2127

Rhode Island
Elder Abuse Hotline
In-State: 800 322-2880
Adult Services
Department of Human Services
Cranston, RI
401 464-2651

Or

Department of Elderly Affairs
Providence, RI
401 277-2858
401 277-2880

South Carolina
Commission on Aging
Columbia, SC
803 735-0210

Or

Division of Adult Services
Office of Children, Family and Adult
Services
Department of Social Services
Columbia, SC
803 734-5670

South Dakota
Office of Adult Services and Aging
Pierre, SD
605 773-3656

Tennessee
Commission on Aging
Nashville, TN
615 741-2056

Or

Protective Services
Social Services Programs
Department of Human Services
Nashville, TN
615 741-5926

Texas
Elder Abuse Hotline
In-State: 800 252-5400
Department on Aging
Austin, TX
512 444-2727

Or

Adult Protective Services
Department of Human Services
Austin, TX
512 450-3211

Utah
Division of Aging and Adult Services
Department of Social Services
Salt Lake City, UT
801 538-3910

Vermont
Elder Abuse Hotline
In-State: 800 564-1612
Commissioner Aging and Disabilities
Waterbury, VT
802 241-2400

Or

Adult Protective Services
Waterbury, VT
802 241-2345

Virginia
Department for the Aging
Richmond, VA
804 225-2271

Or

Protective Services
Bureau of Adult and Family Services
Department of Social Services
Richmond, VA
804 662-9241

Washington
Aging and Adult Services
Administration/Department of Social
and Health Services
Olympia, WA
206 586-3768

Or

Adult Protective Services
Department of Social and Health
Services
Olympia, WA
206 753-5227

West Virginia
Elder Abuse Hotline
In-State: 800 352-6513
Commission on Aging
Charleston, WV
304 558-3317

Or

Services to the Aged, Blind and
Disabled
Social Services Bureau
Department of Human Services
Charleston, WV
304 558-7980

Wisconsin
Bureau of Aging
Division of Community Services
Madison, WI
608 266-2536

Wyoming
Hotline Elder Abuse
In-State: 800 528-3396
Commission on Aging
Cheyenne, WY
307 777-7986

APPENDIX F

Glossary

abrasion   a scraping or rubbing away of surface of the skin by friction.

abuse   improper use of equipment, a substance, or a service such as a drug or program, whether intentionally or unintentionally.

amino acid   an organic chemical compound composed of one or more basic amino groups and one or more of the acidic carboxyl groups.

ammonium ampule   aromatic stimulant used in treating syncope.

anaphylactic shock   severe and sometimes fatal systemic hypersensitivity reaction to a sensitizing substance such as a drug, vaccine, certain food, etc.

angina pectoris   paroxysmal thoracic pain caused most often by myocardial anoxia as a result of atherosclerosis of the coronary arteries.

angiocath   a hollow, flexible tube that is inserted into a blood vessel to withdraw or insert fluid.

anti-social behavior   a behavior that exhibits repetitive behavioral pattern that lacks moral and ethical standards.

aorta   the largest artery, branches off from the heart.

apnea   cessation of breathing.

arterial   pertaining to large blood vessels that carry blood in a direction away from the heart.

assessment   evaluation or appraisal of a condition or situation.

atherosclerosis   arterial disorder characterized by build up of cholesterol, lipids, and cellular debris within large and medium sized arteries.

atropine   an alkaloid that works by blocking the parasympathetic stimuli by raising the threshold of response of effector cell to acetylcholine.

avulsion   the separation by tearing of any part of the body from the whole.

bag valve mask   a manually operated resuscitator that consists of a bag reservoir, a one-way flow valve, and a face mask that is capable of ventilating a non-breathing patient.

bandage   a strip or roll of cloth or other material used to secure a dressing, maintain pressure, or immobilize a part of the body.

Betadine   topical anti-infective (providone-iodine).

burnout   mental or physical energy depletion after a period of chronic, unrelieved job-related stress.

butterfly needle   small needle used most often to start IV solutions. Can be used for phlebotomy.

capillary   the smallest blood vessel.

chain of command   the order in which authority or responsibility of decision making descends through the organization or medical team.

circulatory system   a network of channels through which the nutrient fluids of the body circulate.

CNS   central nervous system consists of the brain and spinal cord.

congestive heart failure   a condition that reflects impaired cardiac action resulting in volume overload.

contraindicated   a factor that prohibits the administration of a drug or procedure for a specific patient with a specific condition.

cyanosis   bluish discoloration of the skin and mucous membrane caused by an excess of deoxygenated hemoglobin in the blood.

diphenhydramine   antihistaminic medication; trade name is Benadryl.

diagnosis   determination of the type and cause of a health condition based on all information gathered.

distress   an emotional or physical state of pain, sorrow, misery, suffering, or discomfort.

documentation   written account of an event.

dressing   a clean or sterile covering applied directly to wounded or diseased tissue.

edema   abnormal accumulation of fluid in the interstitial spaces of the body's tissue.

embolus   a circulating mass in a blood vessel; foreign material that obstructs a blood vessel.

emergency   a serious situation that arises suddenly and threatens the life or welfare of a person or a group of people, as a natural disaster or a medical crisis.

EMS   emergency medical services.

epinephrine   an endogenous adrenal hormone and synthetic adrenergic vasoconstrictor.

eustress   a positive form of stress.

failure to thrive   the abnormal retardation of the growth and development of an infant.

fatty acid   any of the several organic acids produced by the hydrolysis of neutral fat.

flowmeter   device operated by a needle valve in an anesthetic gas machine that measures gases by the speed of flow.

fracture   a traumatic injury to a bone in which the continuity of the tissue of the bone is broken.

general adaptation syndrome   the defense response of the body or the psyche to injury or prolonged stress.

glucose   a simple sugar and a major source of energy found in certain food, especially fruits.

gratuitously   without pay or other compensation.

Health Care Consent Act   allows patients to appoint someone to make their health care decisions if the patient becomes unable to do so.

hemostat   small pointed forceps.

hepatomegaly   an enlarged liver.

hyperglycemia   a greater than normal amount of glucose in the bloodstream, as in diabetes.

hypertension   disorder characterized by elevated blood pressure.

hypoglycemia   a less than normal amount of glucose in the bloodstream.

hypothermia   abnormal and dangerous condition in which the temperature of the body is below 95°.

IgE antibodies   immunoglobulin E—one of the five classes of humoral antibodies produced by the body.

immersion burns   a burn that results by placing a body or part of the body in hot water or other liquid.

immunity   the quality of being insusceptible to or unaffected by a particular disease or condition.

incision   a straight wound (cut) made by knife or sharp object.

insulin   a natural hormone secreted by the beta cells of the islets of Langerhans in the pancreas in response to increased levels of glucose in the blood.

Kussmaul respiration   abnormally deep, very rapid sighing respiration characteristic of diabetic ketoacidosis.

liability   something one is obligated to do or an obligation required to be fulfilled by law, usually financial in nature.

lidocaine   topical or local anesthetic agent.

life-prolonging declaration   a form that directs the physician to pursue any or all life-prolonging procedures.

litigation   carrying on or the contesting of a suit.

living will   a written agreement between a patient and physician to withhold heroic measures if the patient's condition is found to be irreversible.

mast cells   a constituent of connective tissue containing large basophilic granules that contain heparin, serotonin, bradykinin, and histamine.

medical malpractice   the charge of neglect of a physician to his/her agents duties or obligations.

metabolism   the aggregate of all chemical processes that take place in living organisms resulting in growth generation of energy elimination of wastes and other bodily functions.

motor skills   the ability to coordinate body functions that involve movement, including gross motor movement, fine motor movement, and motor planning.

mottled   irregularly mixed colors.

Munchausen's Syndrome   also called pathmimicry, a condition characterized by recurrent pleas for medical treatment and/or hospitalization for an imaginary illness with symptoms that may be acute and resolve upon treatment. Munchausen's syndrome is recurrent behavior.

Munchausen's Syndrome by Proxy   a result if caregiver acts in a manner that causes a child to appear ill, resulting in extensive medical care, testing, hospitalization, or surgery for the child.

nasal cannula   a device for delivering oxygen by way of two small tubes that are inserted into the nares.

nasopharyngeal airway   tubular passage for the movement of air into and out of the lungs, inserted in the nasal passages.

neglect   a condition caused by the guardian failing to provide sufficient physical or emotional care to a dependent person.

nitroglycerine   vasodilator most commonly used in the treatment of angina pectoris.

norepinephrine   vasoconstrictor; a hormone secreted by the adrenal medulla.

oropharyngeal airway   a firm airway tube that is inserted into the mouth of an unconscious patient to prevent the flaccid tongue from blocking the airway.

osteogenesis imperfecta   a genetic disorder involving defective development of the connective tissue. It is inherited as an autosomal dominant trait and is characterized by abnormally brittle and fragile bones that are easily fractured by the slightest trauma.

oxygen deprivation   an abnormally low amount of oxygen in the blood caused by a variety of problems.

pancreas   kidney-shaped, grayish pink nodular gland that stretches transversely across the posterior abdominal wall and secretes various substances such as digestive enzymes, insulin, and glucagon.

parenteral   denotes medication route not in or through the digestive system; injection.

paresthesia   numbness or tingling in parts of the body.

personal protective equipment (PPE)   items such as masks, gloves, aprons, etc. used to prevent the spread of blood-borne pathogens.

pharyngeal wall   the wall of the pharynx located in the throat.

plasma   the watery, straw-colored fluid portion of the lymph and blood.

puncture   a wound or opening made by piercing with a pointed object.

rape   a sexual assault; rape is a crime of violence, and its victims are treated for medical and psychological trauma.

refusal-of-treatment form   the form used to document the refusal of treatment by the patient.

respondeat superior   the concept that an employer may be held liable for torts committed by employees acting within their scope of training.

rigor mortis   a rigid condition of the skeletal and cardiac muscle shortly after death.

sclera   the tough inelastic, opaque membrane covering the posterior five sixths of the eyebulb.

seizure   a hyper-excitation of neurons in the brain.

social skills   the abilities necessary to live in accordance with the expectations and standards of a group or society.

standard of care   a standard for the practice of a profession, an evaluation that serves as a basis for comparison for evaluating similar phenomena or substances.

standing orders   procedures or medications that can be administered in specific circumstances without a written order from the physician because the procedure is designated by the physician as standard for that particular office under those particular circumstances All standing orders must be in writing, signed and dated.

status epilepticus   continual seizures occurring without interruption a true medical emergency.

STD   sexually transmitted disease.

stress   an emotional, physical, social, economic or other factor that requires a response or change.

sudden infant death syndrome (SIDS)   the unexpected and sudden death of an apparently normal and health infant that occurs during sleep and with no physical or autopsy evidence of death.

superficial   of or pertaining to the skin or another surface.

sympathetic nervous system   a division of the autonomic nervous system.

syncope   fainting.

syndrome   a complex of signs and symptoms resulting from common cause or appearing, in combination to present a clinical picture of a disease.

syrup of Ipecac   medication to induce vomiting.

threshold limit   the point at which a psychological or physiological effect begins to be produced.

thrombosis   a blood clot.

TIA   transient ischemic attack—mini strokes leaving no residual effects

tongue blade   wooden or plastic blade used to hold the tongue down when examining the back of the throat.

tourniquet   a device used in controlling hemorrhage, consisting of the application of a wide constricting band to the limb proximal to the site of bleeding.

trauma   physical injury caused by violent or disruptive action; can also be mental or emotionally generated.

triage   a process in which a group of patients is sorted according to their needs for care based on the kind of illness or injury, severity of the problem, and the facilities.

vasoconstriction   of or pertaining to a process, condition, or substance that causes the constriction of blood vessels.

vasodilation   enlargement or dilation of blood vessels.

venous   a large vessel that carries blood in a direction toward the heart.

Venturi mask   a respiratory therapy face mask used for administering a controlled concentration of oxygen to the patient.

verbal orders   the spoken orders a physician gives to his office staff.

Bibliography

Advanced First Aid and Emergency Care. 2nd Edition. American National Red Cross, Washington, DC, 1988.

Better Documentation. Clinical Skillbuilders, Springhouse Corporation, Springhouse, PA, 1992.

Bergeron, J. David. *First Responder.* 3rd Edition. Brady Englewood Cliffs, NJ, 1994.

Caregivers of Young Children: Preventing and Responding to Child Maltreatment. U.S. Department of Health and Human Services, The Circle, Inc., McLean, VA, 1992.

Child Abuse and Neglect—Identifying and Reporting for Public Health Clinics' Staff. Revised Edition. Indiana State Board of Health, Division of Child and Maternal Health, and Indiana Chapter for the Prevention of Child Abuse, Indianapolis, IN, 1988.

Danger Signs and Symptoms. Clinical Skillbuilders, Springhouse Corporation, Springhouse, PA, 1990.

Dernocorur, Kate Boyd. *Streetsense: Communication, Safety, and Control.* 2nd Edition. Prentice Hall, Englewood Cliffs, NJ, 1989.

Diagnostic and Statistical Manual of Mental Disorders. 3rd Edition, revised. American Psychiatric Association, Washington, DC, 1987.

Diagnostic and Treatment Guidelines on Child Physical Abuse and Neglect. American Medical Association, Chicago, IL, 1992.

Diagnostic and Treatment Guidelines on Child Sexual Abuse. American Medical Association, Chicago, IL, 1992.

Emergency Procedures. Clinical Skillbuilders, Springhouse Corporation, Springhouse, PA, 1991.

Feutz-Harter, Sheryl A. *Nursing and the Law.* 4th Edition. Professional Education Systems, Eau Claire, WI, 1991.

Frew, M. A. and Frew, D. R. *Comprehensive Medical Assisting: Competencies for Administrative and Clinical Practice.* F. A. Davis, Philadelphia, PA, 1994.

Fordney, M. T. and Follis, J. J. *Administrative Medical Assisting.* 3rd Edition. Delmar Publishers, Albany, NY, 1993.

Forward, Dr. Susan. *Toxic Parents.* Bantam Books, New York, NY, 1989.

Gelles, Richard J. and Cornell, Claire Pedrick. *Intimate Violence in Families.* 2nd Edition. Sage Publications, Newberry Park, CA, 1990.

Hafen, Brent Q. and Karren, Keith J. *First Aid for Colleges and Universities.* 5th Edition. Allyn and Bacon, Newton, MA, 1993.

Hafen, Brent Q. and Karren, Keith J. *Prehospital Emergency Care and Crisis Intervention.* 4th Edition. Brady Morton Series, Prentice Hall, Englewood Cliffs, NJ, 1993.

Hegner, Barbara R. and Caldwell, Esther. *Nursing Assistant: A Nursing Process Approach.* 7th Edition. Delmar Publishers, Albany, NY, 1995.

HIV/AIDS Legal Project. *A Legal Handbook for Persons Living with HIV Disease in Indiana.* HIV/AIDS Legal Project, Indianapolis, IN, 1993.

Keir, L., Wise, B. A., and Krebs, C. *Medical Assisting, Clinical and Administrative Competencies.* 3rd Edition. Delmar Publishers, Albany, NY, 1993.

Lane, Karen. *Manual of Medical Assisting Practice.* W. B. Saunders, Philadelphia, PA, 1993.

Lewis, Marcia A. and Tamparo, Carol D. *Medical Law, Ethics and Bioethics in the Medical Office.* 3rd Edition. F. A. Davis, Philadelphia, PA, 1993.

Marieb, Elaine N. *Essentials of Human Anatomy and Physiology.* 4th Edition. Benjamin/Cummings, Redwood City, CA, 1994.

Marsh, Peter, ed. *Eye to Eye: How People Interact.* Salem House, Winston Salem, NC, 1991.

Miller, Dean F. *Dimensions of Community Health.* 3rd Edition. W. C. Brown, Dubuque, IA, 1992.

Miller/Keane. *Encyclopedia and Dictionary of Medicine, Nursing, and Allied Health.* 5th Edition, W. B. Saunders, Philadelphia, PA, 1992.

Mitchell, Jeff and Bray, Grady. *Emergency Services Stress—Guidelines for Preserving the Health and Careers of Emergency Services Personnel.* Brady—Prentice Hall, Inc., Englewood Cliffs, NJ, 1990.

Mulochill, Mary Lou. *Human Diseases: A Systemic Approach.* 3rd Edition. Appleton and Lange, Norwalk, CT, 1991.

NiCarthy, Ginny. *Getting Free—A Handbook for Women in Abusive Relationships.* Seal Press, Seattle, WA, 1986.

Nurse's Handbook of Law and Ethics. Springhouse Corporation, Springhouse, PA, 1992.

Parcel, Guy S. *Basic Emergency Care of the Sick and Injured.* 4th Edition. Mosby Publishing, St. Louis, MO, 1990.

Psychosocial Crises. Clinical Skillbuilders, Springhouse Corporation, Springhouse, PA, 1992.

Rapid Assessment. Clinical Skillbuilders, Springhouse Corporation, Springhouse, PA, 1991.

Slaikeu, Karl A. *Crisis Intervention—A Handbook for Practice and Research.* Allyn and Bacon, Newton, MA, 1984.

Stapleton, Edward and Henry, Mark C. *EMT Prehospital Care.* W. B. Saunders, Philadelphia, PA, 1992.

Tamparo, Carol D. and Lewis, Marcia A. *Diseases of the Human Body.* F. A. Davis, Philadelphia, PA, 1994.

Thygerson, Alton L. *The First Aid Book.* 2nd Edition. Prentice Hall, Englewood Cliffs, NJ, 1986.

Van DeGraf, Kent M. and Fox, Stuart W. A. *Concept of Human Anatomy and Physiology.* 3rd Edition. W. C. Brown, Dubuque, IA, 1992.

Walter, John. *An Introduction to the Principles of Disease.* 3rd Edition. W. B. Saunders, Philadelphia, PA, 1992.

Yvorra, James G., ed. *Mosby's Emergency Dictionary: Quick Reference for Emergency Responders.* Mosby-Year Book, St. Louis, MO, 1989.

Index